Community Rehabilitation in Neurology

Rehabilitation should not stop when the disabled person is discharged from hospital, and many neurological patients require ongoing rehabilitation in order to maximize their functional abilities, minimize complications and promote full participation at home and in the community.

This book analyses community rehabilitation needs from many different perspectives, including the views of disabled people, rehabilitation clinicians and service providers. Many examples of community rehabilitation schemes are presented, with evidence for their effectiveness, and case studies are used to highlight the main issues. The authors take an international view, and there are chapters dealing with the disabled child in the community and with neuropsychological rehabilitation.

The first book to examine the growing trend towards community rehabilitation in neurology, it is directed towards all clinicians involved with neurorehabilitation.

Michael P. Barnes is Professor of Neurological Rehabilitation and Co-Director of the Centre for Rehabilitation and Engineering Studies, University of Newcastle upon Tyne, Hunters Moor Regional Neurorehabilitation Centre, Newcastle upon Tyne. He is Founder President of the World Federation for Neurological Rehabilitation, and his previous books include *Upper Motor Neurone Syndrome and Spasticity* (with Garth Johnson, Cambridge University Press, 2001).

Harriet Radermacher is Research Associate in Community Rehabilitation, Hunters Moor Regional Neurorehabilitation Centre, Newcastle upon Tyne.

With contributions from **Peter Rosenbaum** MD FRCP, Professor of Paediatrics, and **Mary Law** PhD OT(Reg), Professor and Associate Dean (Health Sciences) Rehabilitation Science and Co-Director, CanChild Centre for Childhood Disability Research, both of McMaster University, Hamilton, Ontario, Canada; and **Pamela Klonoff** PhD ABPP-CN, Clinical Director and Neuropsychologist, and **David Lamb** PhD ABPP-CN, Neuropsychologist, both of Barrow Neurological Institute, Phoenix, Arizona, USA.

Community Rehabilitation
in Neurology

Michael P. Barnes

and

Harriet Radermacher
Hunter's Moor Regional Neurorehabilitation Centre,
Newcastle upon Tyne

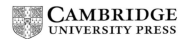

CAMBRIDGE
UNIVERSITY PRESS

PUBLISHED BY THE PRESS SYNDICATE OF THE UNIVERSITY OF CAMBRIDGE
The Pitt Building, Trumpington Street, Cambridge, United Kingdom

CAMBRIDGE UNIVERSITY PRESS
The Edinburgh Building, Cambridge CB2 2RU, UK
40 West 20th Street, New York, NY 10011-4211, USA
477 Williamstown Road, Port Melbourne, VIC 3207, Australia
Ruiz de Alarcón 13, 28014 Madrid, Spain
Dock House, The Waterfront, Cape Town 8001, South Africa

http://www.cambridge.org

First published 2003

Printed in the United Kingdom at the University Press, Cambridge

Typefaces Minion 11/14.5 pt, Formata and Formata BQ   *System* LATEX 2$_\varepsilon$ [TB]

A catalogue record for this book is available from the British Library

Library of Congress Cataloguing in Publication data

Barnes, Michael P., 1952–
Community rehabilitation in neurology / Michael Barnes, Harriet Radermacher.
p.   cm.
Includes bibliographical references and index.
ISBN 0 521 80874 X (hardback)
1. Nervous system – Diseases – Patients – Rehabilitation. 2. Community health services.
I. Radermacher, Harriet, 1975–   II. Title.
[DNLM: 1. Nervous System Diseases – rehabilitation. 2. Community Health Services.
WL 140 B261c 2003]
RC350.4 .B37 2003
616.8′043–dc21   2002031347

ISBN 0 521 80874 X hardback

Contents

Background to community neurological rehabilitation

Why did we want to write this book? There are now many textbooks on rehabilitation, including an increasing number specifically about neurological rehabilitation. However, most of these texts are written from the standpoint of a traditional hospital-based medical speciality. Many, understandably, deal with diseases and symptom management with very little attention paid to the broader concepts of disability and community participation. Many disabled people either never enter hospital or spend only a small proportion of their lives within a hospital rehabilitation unit. Thus, it is ironic that modern rehabilitation practice, at least in the Western world, has a hospital focus. There is a clear need for coordinated rehabilitation to be provided in the home, or at least in the local community. This is a significant gap in health-service provision.

We are not aware of any major review of the literature on community rehabilitation and thus we thought it was an opportune moment to write this book. The expertise of the lead authors is in the field of neurological rehabilitation and so we have generally restricted our comments and critiques to this arena. Our primary aim is to review the need behind the provision of community rehabilitation and address the evidence for the efficacy of such community interventions. We hope this will not only stimulate clinical developments in this field but also encourage further research so that the evidence base may become more robust than at present. We hope that we have succeeded in these aims.

Neurological rehabilitation practice in the developed world (the North in modern parlance) has tended to be hospital focused and has concentrated on assisting disabled people in the postacute phase of their disability. This is the phase that follows in the weeks and months after an acute disabling event, particularly stroke and traumatic brain injury. There has been scant attention to the needs of disabled people after this phase is over and after they have been discharged back home. Modern neurological rehabilitation has often failed to deal with the needs of individuals who never come to the attention of an acute rehabilitation unit, such as those people with cerebral palsy or multiple sclerosis. These people mainly live in the community and only come into contact with rehabilitation practice at the time of a relapse or the appearance of a complication. Many such complications are unnecessary and avoidable if the individual had access to an expert multidisciplinary rehabilitation team throughout their life. It is a pity that rehabilitation has largely become a hospital based speciality as by so doing the longer-term needs of people with neurological disabilities can be overlooked. It is also a pity that community rehabilitation has been perceived as an area into which the health professional should not readily stray. It is certainly true that when disabled people are living at home much of their restriction is not due to their own particular disabilities but to the problems of society. Environmental and attitudinal barriers undoubtedly restrict active participation by disabled people in the local community, in employment, in leisure pursuits and even within their own families. Such societal issues go beyond the expertise of the health professional but surely the clinician has an important role to play in a community setting.

There are indications that health systems are beginning to recognize the longer-term health and rehabilitation needs of disabled people who are living at home. In many countries government resources are beginning to be directed away from acute, and expensive, hospitals towards healthcare delivered within the community. There is more emphasis on the general practitioner and the primary care team. There is also increasing emphasis on initiatives that help support the disabled person within their own home and prevent unnecessary admission to hospital. There are other schemes that facilitate discharge from hospital and support the disabled person after discharge. There are increasing numbers of health professionals who have a remit, either full-time or part-time, to work in the community. We are beginning to see the expert rehabilitation nurse or therapist venturing away from the hospital doors. This is a trend to be encouraged. It is certainly a trend that is entirely compatible with the general views of the disabled people's movement, which has long encouraged a community- and home-based focus for health services.

It is not the purpose of this book to denigrate the hospital-based rehabilitation unit. There is now firm evidence for the efficacy of postacute rehabilitation, particularly in the context of stroke. Such units promote recovery and independence and should be a central component of acute healthcare. In addition to the local hospital rehabilitation unit there is a need for a regional specialist rehabilitation centre, which can cater for the needs of those with the most complex and severe physical and psychological problems. Such centres should act not only as centres of clinical excellence but also as centres of education, training and research for the health community as a whole. More such centres are needed but preferably hand in hand with growth in the community services.

We do not propose the redistribution of scarce rehabilitation resources but hope to make a strong case for increasing such resources overall and directing new energies into community rehabilitation. We would like to see all health professionals working more closely in partnership with disabled people and their families, and other social care professionals, within the community and in the home. However, we are aware that new initiatives in the modern health service need to be firmly evidence based and the main purpose of this book is to review such evidence. We hope this will help others make a stronger case for the development of community initiatives. We are conscious that the quality and quantity of rehabilitation research literature in the community is lacking. It is our intention that by reviewing available literature the gaps in the field will become more apparent and the focus of future research become clearer.

We are conscious that this book concentrates on neurological problems and obviously we are aware that many people in the community have a range of other diagnoses, including cardiac, musculoskeletal and psychiatric problems. However, these areas are outside our field of expertise, although we have referred to other groups where particular examples seem pertinent to the neurological field. Throughout this text we have emphasized that it is inappropriate to differentiate between physical disability and the psychological, behavioural and emotional problems associated with disability. It is vital in a community setting to adopt a holistic view of the disabled person, which clearly needs to encompass the whole spectrum of problems that may be encountered.

A note on language. There is a discrepancy within disability groups in the North about the way in which we should refer to disabled people. In disability groups in America and Canada, and also in professional academic texts in the UK, the preferred term is persons with disabilities. It is based on the people first philosophy – that people come before the disability. However, disability groups in the UK disagree because this implies that the disability is an attribute of the person and not of society. The British social model of disability (see Chapter 3) tends to advocate the use of the term disabled person. We have tried to adopt this approach as far as possible. However, we are aware that the different contexts of the chapters have sometimes required different terminology and we hope not to have caused offence in any chapter by inappropriate use of language. Discussions of semantics should not be to the exclusion of addressing the real issues facing disabled people.

How is the book structured? We have introduced the broad topic of rehabilitation in Chapter 2 with an overview of rehabilitation practice in general and neurological rehabilitation in particular. This chapter introduces the concepts of impairment, disability and handicap as well as the more modern concepts of impairment, activity and participation. In this chapter we review the need for community-based rehabilitation and place this need in the context of the views of disabled people, the developments in the health professions and advances in health systems. We also discuss a number of theoretical models of how community rehabilitation may be delivered in a variety of different settings, from hospital outreach on the one hand to models of independent living on the other.

There has been a tendency in the past for the theoretical constructs of disability to be firmly divided into two camps – the medical model and the social model. These are important concepts for discussion in a textbook of this type and we do so in Chapter 3. However, this chapter also emphasizes the urgent need for more collaboration between the two camps and the need to develop an integrated and dynamic network of partnerships not only between health and social care professionals but also between professionals and the disabled person and their family.

The word community is sometimes used too glibly. The social science literature abounds with various definitions and discussions on the concept of community and these thoughts are put into context in Chapter 4.

The disabled persons' movement now has a long history in many countries, particularly the USA. In that country, and in a few others, it has been instrumental in setting the agenda for rehabilitation services. In many other countries the views of disabled people are now becoming paramount in designing disability services. This is a trend that should be applauded and encouraged. Chapter 5 attempts to summarize and debate the views of disabled people within a community context.

A particular emphasis of this textbook is on the need to develop a firm evidence base that can act as a platform for the development of future services. We are conscious that many people working in the community sector have little, if any, experience of research and we felt it was appropriate to summarize briefly basic research principles and have done so in Chapter 6. In particular we wish to flag some of the difficulties and challenges of working within the community. However, we hope we have not portrayed these challenges as too severe and put people off the important task of developing a more robust research base for neurological rehabilitation in the community. It was certainly not our intention to do so and indeed we hope we have tried to portray some of the interest and excitement that can be generated by simple research or audit projects and the publication and dissemination of such results.

The key chapter in this book is Chapter 7. In this chapter we have tried to review the evidence base for community rehabilitation. This has been a major challenge. There is sparse high-quality peer-review literature on the subject but nevertheless there is a significant array of small-scale research, both quantitative and qualitative, and a wealth of anecdotal experience. We have tried to summarize an extraordinarily complicated field in a tangible and understandable fashion.

Occasionally health professionals in the North forget that their compatriots in the South have been working in the field of community rehabilitation for many years. In less developed countries there are very few hospital-based rehabilitation facilities and the overwhelming majority of disabled people have never accessed and never will access such a unit. Indeed, most disabled people do not have access to any health professional at all. If there is any contact then it has often been through a Community-Based Rehabilitation (CBR) project, which in turn has often been organized, financed and even run by international nongovernmental organizations (NGOs). Many successful and diverse projects have been established and it seemed appropriate for the North to learn some lessons from the South. Chapter 8 serves this purpose. The CBR literature is diverse and often difficult to access but we have tried to pull together some strands that may be of relevance to this textbook.

Naturally, the book has concentrated on health-related matters but throughout the text we have emphasized the need to consider all aspects of community. Chapter 9 discusses employment rehabilitation as well as issues relating to housing, sport and leisure, transport and driving and education. We briefly touch on issues such as alternative therapies and the role of charitable and voluntary agencies as well as emphasizing the need for support of the carers of disabled people, and indeed support to the family as a whole. We are aware that this chapter has to be somewhat parochial as these broader issues depend so much on the local society, local culture and national legislation. However, we hope that we have portrayed at least some of the evidence that emphasizes the importance of these broader aspects of service provision in the community.

The thrust of the book is towards adults. However, there are significant numbers of children with disabilities who live at home and thus we asked Peter Rosenbaum and Mary Law to provide a chapter, which introduces the concepts of childhood disability (Chapter 10). We are very grateful for their insightful contribution.

Many individuals with neurological disabilities have a complicated range of cognitive, intellectual and behavioural problems, in addition to their physical disabilities. This is particularly true for people with traumatic brain injury and many other diseases, such as multiple sclerosis and stroke. Neuropsychologists have been at the forefront of the management of such problems and many models for neuropsychological rehabilitation have now been developed. This is a specialist field and this book does not attempt to offer a definitive guide to neuropsychological rehabilitation. However, we felt it was important to cover this aspect of community rehabilitation in a little more detail. Thus, we asked Pamela Klonoff and David Lamb to summarize some of the initiatives around the field of neuropsychological rehabilitation in the community. They have provided an excellent chapter (Chapter 11), which reviews this literature and draws upon particular examples of practice from their own unit in Phoenix, Arizona.

Illustrative case studies

At this point we felt it might be useful to illustrate some of the difficulties that can occur for people with neurological disabilities without appropriate community rehabilitation and support. Thus, we will briefly annotate four case studies taken from the authors' experience in the northeast of England. For the purpose of illustration these are studies where significant problems have arisen. The studies should not be taken as indicative of the general level of rehabilitation in the northeast! Clearly, many people go through a hospital-based rehabilitation process with an excellent outcome. Sometimes unnecessary problems can arise where there is no community rehabilitation. These case studies will be revisited in Chapter 12. At that point some of the advantages of community rehabilitation will have been illustrated and the literature reviewed. We will then postulate what may have happened if there had been proper community rehabilitation.

Case study 1

Mr B is a 67-year-old retired gardener. He led an active life and had been fully employed as a railway engine driver until his retirement at the end of 65 years. He has been a moderate smoker and has mild hypertension well controlled with prescription of a diuretic. He had been 2 years into active retirement when he had his stroke. Mr and Mrs B have no children. Mrs B has been mildly disabled with cerebral palsy all her life. She has no cognitive impairments but does have a relatively mild left hemiparesis. She is a little older than Mr B and in recent years her walking has become more difficult for her. She has become much less able to get around outside the house, although she still manages to get around inside the house by holding on to furniture. Mr and Mrs B have no immediate family but live in a small ex-mining community in the north of England and have a number of close friends in their locality.

Mr B had a serious stroke, which left him with a profound left hemiparesis as well as left-sided sensory and visual neglect. He required admission to the local acute hospital where he underwent appropriate investigations, which confirmed a right temporoparietal infarct. He remained on the acute ward and over the course of the next 2 weeks he made slow but steady improvement. At this time he had input from physiotherapy and continued to have medical and nursing support but regrettably there was no active, coordinated rehabilitation and no input from occupational therapy or neuropsychology. After 2 weeks he became depressed and was reluctant to participate in rehabilitation and was becoming anxious about his wife who had been left at home. He was concerned about her ability to cope, although she did have support from her neighbours. He began to stay in bed more and on the busy ward his pressure care was less than satisfactory, and regrettably at the end of the third week he developed a small pressure sore in the sacral area that rapidly progressed over the course of the next fortnight. A further complication arose after about 5 weeks when the pressure sore became infected with methicillin-resistant *Staphylococcus aureus* (MRSA). At this point referral was made to the rehabilitation centre and he was eventually transferred a further 3 weeks later (now 2 months poststroke). His rehabilitation was hampered by a significant pressure sore, which took a further 3 months to heal. Over this time he had begun to make a reasonable physical recovery from his left hemiparesis and by the time of his discharge, 6 months poststroke, he was able to walk independently and was independent in all self-care tasks. His left-sided visual and sensory neglect had also largely resolved and he was able to return home and continue looking after his wife.

In total he had been in hospital around 6 months. His wife had managed at home over this period of time but only by resorting to an extensive network of neighbour support.

Case study 2

Mrs W is a 78-year-old lady who is a retired schoolmistress. She lives by herself as her husband died some years previously. She has one son with whom she maintains contact but he lives in London and visits only infrequently. She has no previous medical history and no previous transient ischaemic attacks. However, despite being in good health she had a mild stroke resulting in a right hemiparesis and a degree of dysarthria. Initially her physical disability was relatively mild and she was against going into hospital and thus her general practitioner decided that she be allowed to stay at home. There were, in any case, difficulties in finding her an acute hospital bed.

In the first few days she managed reasonably well and was still just mobile around her home. However, she had difficulty getting to the shops and although she had one or two local friends she was an independent lady who preferred to look after herself and do her own shopping. There was an incline from her house to her local shops and she had great difficulty in getting up this slope. When she did get to the shops she also found communication was awkward because of her dysarthria and she became embarrassed about the slurring of speech.

At some point in the first few days after the stroke she also began to develop trouble-some spasticity and after the first week or so her gait became worse and she was less able, and less willing, to go out of the house by herself. A few weeks after the stroke her gait had slowed further, secondary to the spasticity, and she became occasionally incontinent. The incontinence was probably due to her slowed gait and her difficulty getting to and from the toilet rather than any inherent bladder difficulty. Her general practitioner remained intermittently in touch with her but she had no other rehabilitation support. She became more and more isolated in the home and more dependent on her neighbours. Probably as a result of all these difficulties she became depressed, which in turn further worsened her mobility and her interaction with her friends.

Eventually, around 3 months after the stroke, her general practitioner decided, with her reluctant agreement, that she was no longer able to live at home and she was admitted to a local nursing home.

Case study 3

Mrs M is a 33-year-old lady who has had multiple sclerosis for the last 8 years. Initially she had two relapses over the first 2 years of the illness and then entered a reasonably static phase. Over this time she had a relatively mild spastic paraparesis and a relatively minor degree of urinary frequency and urgency. However, in the previous 2 years she had three further relapses and on each occasion the relapse further weakened her legs and her bladder symptoms. In addition she developed a relatively minor degree of ataxia of the hands and a slight degree of dysarthria. However, in between the relapses she largely reverted to her previous physical state although there was probably a minor over-all worsening of the symptoms. She lives at home with her two daughters aged 10 years and 8 years. She is married but her husband works on the oilrigs in the North Sea and is away from home for several weeks at a time. Her parents have died but she has a sister who lives nearby who has her own family, and although she is able to help out her involvement needs to be minimal. Mrs M worked as a receptionist for a local small business.

At each of the relapses in the last 2 years she had been admitted to the local neurology department for administration of intravenous steroids and physiotherapy but neverthe-less the admissions caused her considerable inconvenience as her children then needed to be looked after by her sister and Mrs M needed several days off work. Her employer dismissed her after her most recent relapse. Mrs M is currently taking this employer to an industrial tribunal for unfair dismissal but at the moment remains out of work.

Case study 4

Mr Y is a 23-year-old man who at the time of his accident was living at home with his parents. He was unemployed. He was the driver of a car that was involved in a collision with a lamp-post and as a result of the impact Mr Y had a severe traumatic brain injury. He had a few minutes of retrograde amnesia and around 3 days of posttraumatic amnesia (PTA). He was admitted from the scene of the accident to the neurosurgical department but did not require any neurosurgical intervention. He was monitored over the course of 10 days or so as he emerged from coma and PTA and about 2 weeks after his accident was transferred to the local regional head-injury rehabilitation centre. At that stage it was clear that he had made quite a good physical recovery from his injuries and was only left with a mild left hemiparesis, which was of very little functional significance.

The situation, however, was complicated by his severe behavioural problems. He be-came easily physically and verbally aggressive to the staff. The situation was compounded by difficulties with recent memory, poor concentration, impaired information-processing speed and consequent difficulties of both learning about and cooperating with a reha-bilitation programme designed to assist his behavioural problems. He needed constant prompting, guidance and supervision. The neuropsychologist at the centre, with the support of the nursing and therapy staff, put together an active behavioural rehabilitation regime. However, Mr Y consistently failed to cooperate with the programme. His parents were also rather antagonistic to the programme and wished him to be discharged home. Considerable effort was expended in trying to assist Mr Y with the behavioural regime. Further efforts were made to explain the nature of his problems to his parents. However, little progress was possible and after about four weeks on the brain injury unit Mr Y took his own discharge against medical advice, with the assistance and cooperation of his parents. However, his problems, not surprisingly, continued while he was at home. The home situation was fraught and his parents were finding it increasingly difficult to cope with his behavioural problems. After about a further month they decided they could not cope any more and Mr Y moved into his girlfriend's house. She already had a young child and the situation became even more fraught as Mr Y was verbally aggressive, but fortunately not physically aggressive, towards both his girlfriend and the small baby. Eventually this situation broke down and Mr Y moved into a local hostel for homeless men. At this point he began to drift into crime and was eventually arrested for taking a vehicle without the owner's consent. Mitigating circumstances of his head injury were pleaded by some of the staff from the regional head-injury centre and Mr Y did not receive a custodial sentence. After this he decided to move out of the area and moved to London to live with his brother. No further details are available.

Readers are invited to bear these case studies in mind throughout the book. We make some suggestions for how these situations could have been avoided in Chapter 12 but the reader will no doubt develop alternative ideas about how these unfortunate scenarios could have been prevented by appropriate community rehabilitation.

In summary, we hope this book addresses the need to develop rehabilitation services within the community and summarizes the current evidence base for the efficacy of such services. This case is not made in an attempt to pull resources away from the hospital rehabilitation unit but is made as a case to increase resources, services and facilities into the field of rehabilitation as a whole. We firmly believe that community rehabilitation is part of an integrated and dynamic network of services. The artificial boundaries between health and social care are blurred and should become more blurred so that the focal point for resources becomes the disabled person.

2

Neurological rehabilitation – basic principles and models of delivery

Introduction

The purpose of this chapter is to place neurological rehabilitation in a historical context and outline some of the basic underlying principles. Neurological rehabilitation is a relatively new subject and has grown up in a hospital-orientated environment. The need for a new community emphasis will be explored and some theoretical models of delivery discussed. However, first it is important to review briefly the epidemiology of disability in order for the importance of this subject to be placed in an appropriate context.

Epidemiology

The roots of neurology lie in late nineteenth century psychiatry but over the years a rather false distinction has slowly been made between neurological disorders and psychiatric disorders, even though many important disorders such as schizophrenia, manic-depressive illness and senile dementia almost certainly involve an organic disturbance of brain function. In recent years the false distinction between neurology and psychiatry has been made more apparent by the emergence of neurological rehabilitation units in which it is increasingly recognized that the clear distinction is unhelpful. People with traumatic brain injury will nearly always have a combination of physical, psychological, emotional and behavioural problems, which require the expertise of a full multidisciplinary team and one that is preferably trained in both the physical and psychological consequences of disease and injury. Many rehabilitation specialists now also have some training in psychiatry and increasing help is given by the emerging speciality of neuropsychiatry. The importance of the recognition of psychological consequences of disability as

Table 2.1. Incidence and prevalence of neurologically disabling disorders in the UK

Disorder	Incidence per 100 000 population per annum	Prevalence of people with disability per 100 000 population
Cerebral palsy	3^a	200
Cerebral tumour	~15	~30
Dystonia	2–4	24
Encephalitis	~20	?
Epilepsy	~75	500
Guillain-Barré	1	~8
Migraine	–	~500–600
Motor neurone disease	1–2	6
Multiple sclerosis	3–5	100
Muscular dystrophy	~1	4
Parkinson's disease	18–20	150–200
Spina bifida	$2–3^a$	?
Stroke	200	300
Syringomyelia	?	8
Traumatic brain injury	100–150	100–150
Traumatic spinal cord injury	1–2	~80

^{a} Per 1000 live births.

well as the physical consequences is stressed throughout this book. However, in terms of epidemiology this text concentrates on 'classical' neurological problems.

There is a further unhelpful distinction between neurological disorders giving rise to physical disability and other neurological disorders that similarly give rise to an intermittent disturbance of function (e.g. epilepsy) or disorders that simply cause pain (e.g. trigeminal neuralgia and migraine). Services for the latter two groups are often ignored when planning rehabilitation services despite the fact that the prevalence of epilepsy and migraine exceed the prevalence of all other neurologically disabling disorders put together (see Table 2.1).

Around 80% of the diagnostic categories of people admitted into a neurological rehabilitation service are covered by the three leading causes of disability in the Western world – stroke, traumatic brain injury and multiple sclerosis.

Stroke

The incidence of stroke is around two per 1000 population per annum. Around one-third of these people will die within the first month, another third will recover completely without the need for rehabilitation intervention, which leaves around a further third who are likely to survive with a residual disability. It is obviously the latter population that are the main candidates for rehabilitation (Oxfordshire Community Stroke Project, 1983). Most individuals with stroke are admitted to hospital and there is an increasing tendency for such people to be either admitted acutely or transferred soon after admission to a dedicated stroke unit. There is now excellent evidence of the efficacy of stroke units in terms of improved outcome (Langhorne et al., 1993 and *vide infra*). People who survive stroke with a residual disability clearly have a number of major ongoing rehabilitation needs both while in hospital and later in the community. The prevalence of individuals who have had a stroke is around 600 per 100 000 population and roughly half of these people (i.e. 300 per 100 000 population) will have a residual significant disability (Wade and Langton-Hewer, 1987). Individuals can be left with a whole range of difficulties, particularly problems with mobility, self-care and communication, and often a number of cognitive and emotional problems, such as difficulty with memory, perception and depression. The majority of survivors of stroke eventually return home, which in turn gives rise to further pressures on the family and main carers.

Overall, it is estimated that around one-quarter of all severely disabled people living in the community have had a stroke (Langton-Hewer, 1993).

Traumatic brain injury

Admission to hospital as a result of brain injury is remarkably common and it is estimated that about 250–300 people are admitted per 100 000 population per year (British Society of Rehabilitation Medicine 1998). Many people with a mild traumatic brain injury are admitted only briefly to the casualty department or kept overnight and discharged home. The longer-term problems of mild head injury should not be underestimated but most effort in terms of neurological rehabilitation is directed towards those with more severe brain injury. Around 10–15 people per 100 000 population per year are likely to be left with a permanent and severe disability as a result of traumatic brain injury. As long-term survival is often not impaired the prevalence of people with an ongoing disability is reasonably high, and the best estimates indicate there are 100–150 individuals with a persistent disability per 100 000 population. Brain injury provides a major challenge to a rehabilitation team as there is often a wide variety of physical, psychological, emotional and behavioural problems with major impact not only on the person with the head injury but their wider family. There is ample evidence that the main problems following brain injury are related to family, social and community reintegration and occur after discharge from a postacute rehabilitation unit (Oddy et al., 1985).

Multiple sclerosis

Multiple sclerosis (MS) is the most disabling neurological condition to occur in the young adult population. The incidence is around 3–5 per 100 000 population per year. The prevalence is known to vary significantly according to distance from the equator. Even within the relatively small size of the UK the prevalence will vary from around 80 per 100 000 on the south coast to up to 150 per 100 000 in northern Scotland. The average prevalence is around 120 per 100 000. The majority of individuals will have at least some form of disability and it is likely that everybody will benefit from some input from an informed rehabilitation team, at least in terms of education and advice. Unfortunately, many postacute neurological rehabilitation units do not admit people with multiple sclerosis as they will never present to the acute hospital service. Thus, the availability of rehabilitation varies from district to district, particularly in terms of long-term community support. However, the need for access to a skilled multidisciplinary team is becoming more important as evidence emerges of the efficacy of such input (*vide infra*) as well as the increasing need to access disease-modifying drugs, such as steroids and interferons. In a similar fashion to brain injury, multiple sclerosis can present with a wide and often bewildering variety of physical symptoms as well as cognitive and emotional problems.

Parkinson's disease

Parkinson's disease is the commonest form of disability in older life. The incidence is thought to be around 18–20 per 100 000 population per year with a prevalence of around 150–200 per 100 000 population. The disorder becomes more common as age progresses and approximately one in 10 people over the age of 80 have Parkinsonism. However, the mean age of onset is 55 years and thus the disorder is not exclusively a problem of the elder person and will often occur in individuals who are still economically active. Although Parkinson's disease and other forms of parkinsonism can often be effectively treated in the early years of the disorder, control becomes increasingly difficult and complex in later stages. As the disease progresses a wide variety of other problems can emerge, which clearly need the input of a multidisciplinary rehabilitation team. People with Parkinson's disease do not often have acute presentations and thus will often miss out on the services provided by hospital-based rehabilitation units. In a number of different countries community-based Parkinson's disease teams are now emerging, often under the guidance of a geriatrician. Physiotherapy, occupational therapy and speech therapy input are particularly important in the context of later-stage Parkinson's disease.

Cerebral palsy

Precise epidemiological figures regarding the incidence and prevalence of cerebral palsy are difficult to come by and often vary significantly. A figure of around three individuals with cerebral palsy per 1000 live births is often quoted (Rosen and Dickinson, 1992). The majority of individuals who survive the first few days after birth live a reasonably normal life span, but often with a potentially wide variety of physical and learning difficulties. Thus, there is a reasonably high prevalence of disabling cerebral palsy in the community – perhaps around 200 per 100 000 population. While people with cerebral palsy are still children there is usually a range of support through the educational and social service sectors, often with the involvement of an appropriate paediatric team. However, difficulties commonly arise at school-leaving age when the paediatric and educational services are left behind and the individual passes into a health and social system that is not geared to their needs and often fails to recognize those needs in the young adult. A generic disability team in a given locality may support some young people but people with cerebral palsy will have no ongoing support from the health system and will often present when unnecessary complications have arisen. Problems with spasticity, muscle contracture, wheelchairs, ill-fitting orthoses, pressure sores, communication problems and incontinence are common (Bax et al., 1998). The reader is referred to Chapter 10 on this subject by Peter Rosenbaum and Mary Law.

Traumatic spinal cord injury

The incidence of traumatic spinal cord injury is relatively low, at about 1–2 per 100 000 population per annum. Some individuals will make a full recovery but most are left with residual disability. As traumatic spinal cord injury tends to occur in a younger age group and as survival is now reasonably normal (except for those with very high cervical cord lesions), the prevalence is correspondingly high at around 80 per 100 000 population. It is interesting to note that in many countries, particularly the UK, there is an excellent network of spinal cord injury centres that supports this population both acutely and often in the longer term. Follow-up is generally well organized and long-term complications thus often avoided. While the spinal injury network provides an excellent service it is ironic that many more people with other equally disabling neurological conditions have been largely ignored in the longer term by health and social services.

Other disabling disorders

Naturally there are a wide variety of other neurological problems that can cause short- and long-term disability. Epilepsy and migraine have been mentioned as being the leading disorders in terms of prevalence, but in most parts of the world these disorders are firmly in the province of the acute neurologist and it is unusual for there to be longer-term community support. However, these disorders can both be disabling and can give the individual significant problems with work and home life.

The danger of focusing on diagnostic labels is that services could be established for such groups (e.g. a community MS team), which will then ignore the needs of those with equally severe and disabling problems but with a different diagnostic label. The prevalence of other disabling neurological disorders may be smaller but the needs of other populations can be just as diverse. Motor neurone disease, cerebral tumour, syringomyelia, Guillain–Barré syndrome, dystonia, muscular dystrophy and the after-effects of meningitis/encephalitis are all examples of other neurological entities that will clearly cause significant disability in the long term.

Most of the epidemiology in the neurological arena has been focused on disease entities. There has been relatively little work focusing on generic symptoms. This is mainly because the health field is used to working in disease-related areas. In some ways there is relevance in looking at specific diseases as the needs of that population tend to be similar. However, the disadvantage of planning services purely by disease is that individuals with rarer diseases will tend to be marginalized. In addition, an alternative way of planning services is to organize around particular problems such as spasticity or continence. To an individual who has spasticity it does not really matter whether the cause is head injury, spinal injury, multiple sclerosis or another disease state. Regrettably, there are few epidemiological data that help plan services from the point of view of the disability domains. The only thorough work in the UK was the national census undertaken by the Office of Population Censuses and Surveys (OPCS), which reported in 1988 and 1989. This was a significant survey of the population and made a valuable contribution to our knowledge of disability. The survey found that the prevalence of overall disability among adults was 135 per 1000 population (age 16 years and over). If people living in institutions were included the prevalence increased to 142 per 1000 population. The survey identified 13 different types of disability (Table 2.2). Difficulty with locomotion was the most common problem and had the highest prevalence of all age groups. Not surprisingly people who were most disabled had combinations of physical and/or sensory and/or mental disabilities (Table 2.3). The OPCS survey developed a useful 10-point category of disability ranging from 0 (mildly disabled) to 10 (severely disabled). While these figures are of interest it is difficult to plan services on the basis of these figures, particularly when the health service remains disease orientated rather than disability orientated.

There are a wide variety of conditions that give rise to long-term neurological disability. In general terms the conditions that present acutely, particularly traumatic brain injury, spinal cord injury and stroke, are reasonably well catered for in terms of acute management. Many hospitals also now have a postacute rehabilitation facility, particularly for people with stroke, although support for other acute neurological problems remains patchy and uncoordinated. As we have seen, the majority of neurological problems give rise to long-term disability and thus there is an obvious need for long-term health and social information, support and advice. Many people, particularly those

Table 2.2. Disability domains – estimates of prevalence of disability in Great Britain by type (ICIDH) and age per 1000 population

Type of disability	Age group			
	16–59	60–74	75+	All adults
Locomotion	31	198	496	99
Hearing	17	110	328	59
Personal care	18	99	313	57
Dexterity	13	78	199	40
Seeing	9	56	262	38
Intellectual function	20	40	109	34
Behaviour	19	40	152	31
Reaching and stretching	9	54	149	28
Communication	12	42	140	27
Continence	9	42	147	26
Disfigurement	5	18	27	9
Eating, drinking and digesting	2	12	30	6
Consciousness	5	10	9	5

Source: Martin et al., 1988.

Table 2.3. Types of disability by severity category expressed as a percentage within each severity group

Type of disability	Severity %					
	1–2	3–4	5–6	7–8	9–10	Total
Other disability (not physical)	38	26	17	5	0	23
Physical	39	35	31	25	18	33
Physical and sensory	21	31	30	36	28	28
Physical and mental (+/− sensory)	2	8	24	34	56	18

with nonprogressive disorders, such as cerebral palsy, or slowly progressive disorders, such as multiple sclerosis, never have access to the rehabilitation team. If a local community-based rehabilitation team exists then there may be other problems of access, such as age, diagnosis or symptom-related referral criteria. There are significant numbers of long-term neurologically disabled people in the community (Table 2.1) who receive no advice or support from the health or social sector.

Brief history of rehabilitation

It is not appropriate in a book of this nature to discuss the development of rehabilitation in detail. However, it is probably relevant to note some of the historical developments that have occurred in the field, particularly in recent years, in order to understand the context for the development of institutional rehabilitation and the relative lack of progress in the field of community rehabilitation. Ironically, given the emphasis of modern rehabilitation, the care of disabled people in the past was embedded in the local community. In the UK the community emphasis was enshrined in the Poor Law in 1601. This law made compulsory for each parish to provide for the poor and disabled people of the parish by levying a rate on all occupiers of property within its boundaries. A parish officer was appointed in order to ensure relief was expended on the 'aged and infirm'. Individuals who moved from one parish to another could be refused help in any parish other than their own. Various amendments to the Poor Law were made in subsequent centuries but a major change came in the recommendation of a Royal Commission in 1834. It recommended that parishes should combine into unions large enough to make feasible the provision of separate workhouses for the infirm as well as the able-bodied. This was the start of the institutional focus for disabled people. The Poor Law continued to operate in the UK until after the Second World War. Although local authorities still retained some statutory provision for services for disabled people (e.g. the Chronically Sick and Disabled Persons Act 1970 and the Disabled Persons Act 1986), most of the health care (not rehabilitation) for disabled people rested with the newly created National Health Service (NHS). In the 1950s to 1980s there was virtually no community provision of services for disabled people and if individuals were not able to look after themselves or be looked after by their family at home then there was little option but admission to a residential home. A number of charitable bodies established large residential institutions to accommodate such disabled people (e.g. the Leonard Cheshire Foundation). From the Second World War there were a few charismatic individuals who pioneered the development of rehabilitation (e.g. Sir Ludwig Guttman at Stoke Mandeville Hospital for people with spinal injuries). However, there was no coordinated government development of the field until the 1980s. The medical speciality of rehabilitation medicine was recognized as a distinct medical speciality in the UK only in 1990. At that point there were a handful of medical doctors specializing in the field. The recognition as a speciality enabled a proper training programme to be established for junior doctors and a decade later there are around 100 consultants in rehabilitation medicine in the UK. Other countries in Europe, the USA, Canada and Australia have also seen a similar growth of the medical speciality over broadly the same timescale. At the same time there has been a growth of specialism in the therapy and nursing professions. As rehabilitation units slowly became established then therapists working in such units were able to specialize. Rehabilitation nursing also became a recognized entity. Growth has been slow and recruitment is still difficult in many fields but nevertheless neurological rehabilitation is now definitely recognized as a valid specialism in the medicine, therapy, psychology and nursing domains. Many professional groups now have their own special interest organization. International recognition is now becoming established, particularly after the formation of the World Federation for Neurological Rehabilitation, which has over 3000 members worldwide and holds an international congress every 3 years. Academic credibility has been slower to develop and there are still very few recognized academic neurological rehabilitation centres in the world. However, progress in academia is slowly developing and the evidence base for rehabilitation is expanding – and indeed the evidence base for community rehabilitation is summarized in this book.

Although the speciality has grown, however, the focus has clearly been on the hospital and institutional orientation in a postacute setting. This has been for a number of reasons. The number of professionals with an interest in the subject has been limited and thus there is a tendency for such individuals to group together in regional centres and provide services to a larger population base. Many of the professionals working in the field were already working in a hospital setting and tended to regroup themselves in the same environment. In addition the demand on rehabilitation services was initially, and to an extent still is, from the acute hospital specialities, to take people from the acute beds into a rehabilitation environment in order to allow for another acute patient to be admitted. Frankly, many rehabilitation units have developed in order to relieve the 'bed blocking' situation in the acute hospitals. More recently, the accumulating evidence base for the efficacy of stroke rehabilitation units has further emphasized the need to develop hospital-based stroke units, which have sometimes grown into more general rehabilitation units. Whilst this is entirely desirable this has meant that limited available resources have been directed into the hospital setting rather than into the community setting. Finally, the speciality has developed important links with other relevant specialisms, such as neurology, rheumatology, orthopaedics, plastic surgery, etc., which in turn are hospital based. Such links have simply further encouraged the growth of rehabilitation as a hospital-based speciality. The medical model (see Chapter 3) has tended to prevail in all rehabilitation units both in the UK and abroad and this emphasis on 'normality' and 'cure' has further tended to encourage the speciality to develop a hospital focus where such a model feels more comfortable and familiar to staff.

On the contrary side there has been limited interest and resource in community rehabilitation. Until recently the majority of health-service resources were placed with hospitals and specialist units and community services were traditionally seen as a rather poor relation. General practitioners had busy workloads and, with a few very notable exceptions, were not able to take the time and interest in people with physical disabilities; there were virtually no medical consultants who had sessions in the community with the exception of a few pioneering individuals in community paediatrics. Services within the home were largely seen as the provision of the local authority social service departments – particularly for the provision of aids and appliances and for personal care support. The fact that, in general, support services for disabled people were split between the local authority for home services and the NHS for hospital services only served to emphasize and widen the gap between hospital and community.

More recently the situation has begun to change. There is an increasing emphasis on primary health care. In the UK much of the health commissioning is now undertaken by primary care trusts with a board of management consisting largely of general practitioners and community health workers. This is slowly ensuring a greater emphasis on community health provision, although not necessarily on provision of services for people with physical disabilities. At the same time there is increasing pressure on hospitals to reduce costs (a global phenomenon) and there has been increasing, albeit small-scale, investment in community health services. Governments are beginning to realize the artificial distinction between social services and health services, and in many parts of Europe governments are now actively supporting the concept of 'joined-up thinking' with the provision of a single budget for community health and social services. More practitioners, particularly nurses, are now employed to work in the community and many are taking a special interest in people with disabilities. In particular the nursing profession has now developed the concept of nurse practitioners, who are senior nurses with additional specialized training in particular fields. In physical disability there are now over 100 MS specialist nurses in the UK as well as a range of specialist nurses in Parkinson's disease, stroke, dystonia, head injury and related fields such as diabetes and people in need of kidney dialysis. Many of these innovations are discussed in later chapters of this book. The medical profession in terms of consultants in rehabilitation medicine has been rather slower to move towards the community. This is partly due to small numbers in the field and the inability to dilute time across many different communities, but also because training still places heavy emphasis on the hospital-based aspects of the speciality. A few new community-based specialists are now being appointed or at least shared between hospital and community.

Finally, there is the increasing influence of disabled people themselves and their peer groups. The disability movement across most of Europe has been relatively underactive, at least compared with colleagues in the USA. However, the disabled peoples' lobby now has an increasingly strong voice and also one that is heard and listened to in governmental and health circles. The clear view of disabled people for provision of services in a community and home setting and the need to provide such services through a social model of disability has now been firmly established. There is more discussion about the views of disabled people in this context in Chapter 5.

In summary, the field of rehabilitation has been slow to develop not only in the UK but also across the world. In most countries the speciality is now a recognized entity but still most rehabilitation professionals work in a post-acute hospital setting. Whilst this provides a valuable service to some disabled people, particularly those who have recently had a stroke or head injury, this development does mean that most disabled people are marginalized and do not have access to any form of rehabilitation team. The political situation is changing, with an increased emphasis on community in many countries and consequently increased resources and professionals with a specific remit to work in the community. In addition to the political and economic drivers towards the community there is an increasing evidence base for both the need to provide such services and the efficacy of such services. This book addresses and discusses this evidence base.

Basic principles of rehabilitation

Rehabilitation has a number of features which differentiate it from other specialities. It is a process that is based on education. It is a process in which the disabled person and family must be involved for it to have any real meaning. Rehabilitation has to go beyond the narrow confines of physical disease and must address both the psychological consequences of disability and the social milieu in which the disabled person has to operate. Rehabilitation is essentially a team process. It is certainly a process that cannot be carried out by physicians alone and requires active partnership with a whole range of other health and social service professionals as well as the disabled person and their family.

Modern rehabilitation practice is based around the concepts of impairment, disability and handicap, as outlined by the World Health Organization in 1980 in the *International Classification of Impairments, Disabilities and Handicaps* (ICIDH) (WHO, 1980). This fundamental concept has recently been redrafted in the form of a new classification of impairments, activities and participation. However, as the old classification is so well known it is worth reviewing both classifications.

Impairment is a descriptive term. It says nothing about the consequence. A right hemiparesis or a left-sided proprioceptive sensory loss are impairments. Whilst these descriptions may be an essential part of the diagnostic process they are of limited value in terms of rehabilitation. Rehabilitation goes beyond impairment and indeed places impairment within the functional context – which is termed disability. There is not always a clear relationship between impairment and consequent disability. As an example, a right hemiparesis (an impairment) can lead at one extreme to a complete inability to walk and at the other extreme only causes some occasional difficulty whilst walking, for instance, over rough ground. It is the disability that matters to the individual and not the impairment. Handicap places the disability into a social context. Inability to walk over rough ground, for example, could be a major problem for a gardener and may preclude employment. However, for an older person living a quiet life at home such disability may present no limitation to the desired lifestyle. Rehabilitation is largely concerned with disability and handicap.

The older classification has been much criticized by disabled people. Many disabled groups have felt the underlying paradigm of the ICIDH is the sick role and the medicalization of disability. The terms disability and handicap in themselves imply a disadvantage and a deviation from the norm (Pfeiffer, 2000). Against this background the WHO has been developing a new classification known as the ICIDH-2 (WHO, 1999). This classification avoids 'handicapist' language and moves more towards a social model of disability. It is still criticized by many groups (Bury, 2000) but nevertheless is an improvement in terms of language and emphasis from the older version. The ICIDH-2 is a multipurpose classification system. It aims to provide a scientific basis for understanding and studying the functional states associated with health conditions as well as aiming to establish a common language for describing such states. It is hoped that it will allow collection of comparative data across countries, healthcare disciplines and different services as well as providing a systematic coding system for universal health information systems. In the new classification the term impairment still exists. This dimension (the body dimension) now comprises two classifications – one for functions of body systems and one for body structure. Basically there is little change with the original concept of impairment. However, disability is now termed the activities dimension and this covers the complete range of activities performed by an individual. Handicap is replaced by the term participation and this dimension classifies areas of life in which the individual is involved, has access to and/or for which there are societal opportunities or barriers. In addition the classification gives a list of environmental factors, which form an integral part of the classification. The new classification was only adopted in 2001 and it is too early to say whether this new version provides a better system of classification than the previous model. The new classification has not altered the fact that rehabilitation works in the domains of activities and participation whereas standard medical practice works in the domain of impairment.

What is the essence of rehabilitation? It can be defined as an active and dynamic process by which a disabled person is helped to acquire knowledge and skills in order to maximize physical, psychological and social function. It should be a process that maximizes functional ability and participation. There are three basic rehabilitation approaches:

- Approaches to reduce disability.
- Approaches designed to acquire new skills and strategies, which will reduce the impact of disability.
- Approaches that help to alter the environment, both physical and social, so that a given disability carries with it as little as possible associated problem of participation in society as a whole.

Rehabilitation in a postacute environment will largely focus on the activity dimension whereas rehabilitation in a community setting will focus more on promoting participation. The boundaries are obviously not clearcut but the distinction is important.

The rehabilitation process

The key to the process of rehabilitation, whether hospital-based or community-based, is the central involvement of the disabled person. This individual, usually with the family, must be fully involved in the process at all times. Preferably the individual should work with the rehabilitation staff to set appropriate goals. Only in this way can the goals seem relevant and important to the person. Ideally individuals should set rehabilitation goals themselves but in some circumstances will need assistance. Perhaps their goals are unrealistically optimistic or sometimes unrealistically pessimistic. Sometimes the individual has such a degree of cognitive impairment or behavioural disturbance that full participatory involvement in the goal-setting process is simply not achievable. In those circumstances key family members and the main carers should be involved, or at least people who know the interests and background of the person. Once this principle is established then rehabilitation goals need to be set. Usually there are at least two and often three stages of goal planning. The first stage is the long-term goal in a postacute rehabilitation setting, for example, the long-term goal could be discharge to home, able to manage stairs and independent in self-care. Often the focus of the hospital unit will be the discharge home. In the community setting the longer-term goals will obviously have a different emphasis. Such goals in the community could be, for example, going out to a familiar pub at least once a week. It could be walking independently in the local neighbourhood for at least half a mile each day. It could be returning to work or finding a new occupation. It could be reducing dependence on a carer, such that the carer is able to get out by him/herself for at least an hour each day. The types of goals are myriad but each one must be seen to be relevant and desirable to the persons involved. It is often appropriate to set one or at least very few long-term goals at a time, otherwise the rehabilitation efforts may be too diffuse. Once the long-term goal or goals have been set then medium- and/or short-term subgoals need to be established so that progress towards the eventual long-term goal can be monitored. If the long-term goal is to walk unaided for at least half a mile around the locality each day in a 3-month period then appropriate subgoals could be set at, for example, fortnightly intervals. These goals could be, perhaps, walking a hundred yards or so down the road with a carer, then withdrawing the carer so the individual manages a few hundred yards by themselves, and then that distance could be slowly built up at appropriate intervals until the long-term goal is achieved. It is essential to set subgoals at realistically short intervals so that progress is monitored and the medium- and long-term goals can be adjusted as necessary. Achievement of shorter-term goals also serves to encourage all concerned that some progress is being maintained.

It is important to emphasize certain parameters that define an appropriate goal. A useful acronym is SMART. The goals should be Sensible, Measurable, Achievable, Relevant and Time-limited. The setting of goals implies an appropriate measurement instrument in order to monitor progress. There are many such outcome measures in use, particularly in a hospital setting, but there are some that can be used in a longer-term and community setting. These are reviewed in Chapter 6. All goals should be measurable. The example above regarding walking distance outside the home is objectively measurable. Subjective opinion is important but is more difficult to measure and purely subjective outcomes are probably best avoided. However, the combination of objectivity and subjectivity is perfectly valid if, for example, a goal is to get out to the pub and socialize for a couple of hours at least once a week. This is objectively measurable. However, the quality of the social interaction in the pub is more difficult to measure but is clearly an important outcome for the person. If the individual goes to the pub and is ignored by old colleagues and friends then this is clearly a poor outcome. Objectivity and subjectivity should go hand in hand.

The other central component of the rehabilitation process is the multidisciplinary rehabilitation team. Very occasionally the disabled person working with a single-discipline therapist can achieve a rehabilitation goal. However, the great majority of goals, particularly in a more varied community setting, will often require multidisciplinary input. Indeed it is vital that goals are set that are relevant to the person and not set according to individual disciplines. It is entirely wrong to set, for example, physiotherapy goals, nursing goals and occupational therapy goals. It is important that all disciplines participate in the goal-setting process and understand the whole range of goals for that individual. It may, for example, be important for the physiotherapist to communicate with the disabled person in a particular fashion that has been established in collaboration with the speech and language therapist. Conversely, it may be important for the speech and language therapist to assist the individual to a chair or towards a table in an appropriate fashion that has been discussed with the physiotherapist. In other words, in a proper rehabilitation process there is no room for artificial, single-discipline boundaries. Individuals will bring their own skills and knowledge to the process according to their qualifications and background but must be prepared to work outside traditional professional boundaries. In a community setting it is very likely that fewer disciplines will be involved than in a postacute setting. Thus, it becomes even more important for one discipline to discuss appropriate goals with other disciplines, even if those disciplines are not able to give much personal time to the individual concerned. It is often necessary for the key contact rehabilitationist to effectively become a generic rehabilitation worker. Such an individual should have a broad understanding of the whole rehabilitation process and at least a fundamental grasp of other disciplines. A few rehabilitation units have now formalized the role of generic rehabilitation assistants who work across professional boundaries and work with the disabled person and their family to deliver cross-discipline rehabilitation goals. These individuals will often work under the guidance and supervision of individual therapists and nurses who may have been initially involved in the goal setting and management process. Regrettably, no nationally recognized formal training for such individuals yet exists.

Virtually all rehabilitation teams who have to deal with people with neurological disabilities need the full complement of professional advice and support. This should include physiotherapy, occupational therapy, speech and
language therapy, clinical psychology, nursing and rehabilitation medicine
input. Occasionally other disciplines will be involved such as social workers,
vocational trainers, counsellors, continence advisors, etc. There is probably
no community-based team that has full-time involvement of all the necessary
individuals and most teams will have to manage with part-time input from
many disciplines, or even no input at all. Obviously this makes the delivery of
effective rehabilitation difficult and emphasizes the need for broader-based
generic training. There are now a few 'transitional rehabilitation' teams or
units. These teams will often specialize in the social, community and employment reintegration of brain-injured people once they have returned home
or in the stage before they are able to return home. These units now tend to
have a number of care workers who work with a few individuals and who
are able to deliver cross-discipline rehabilitation goals with limited specialist
professional advice and support. Regrettably, at least in the UK, most such
transitional units are in the private sector and clients are often funded by
legal settlements.

It is now becoming more common for case managers to be attached to
individual clients. The interpretation of case management varies widely but
it is generally accepted that case management involves the coordination of
a range of different professional inputs to a particular individual. The case
manager may be involved, for example, in the planning and goal-setting
process and may then be responsible for organizing the appropriate care or
therapeutic inputs. They may then supervise the rehabilitation programme
and be responsible, with the client, for adjusting and monitoring the rehabilitation goals. Once again it is regrettable that case management is generally
only available in the private sector and is normally funded by those who have
private means or are involved in legal settlements.

A concept related to the generic worker is the emergence of the nurse
practitioner. These individuals are usually senior and experienced nurses
who develop a particular interest in a given subject. There are now recognized training programmes for nurse practitioners in the fields of multiple
sclerosis, Parkinson's disease, stroke and dystonia as well as disability-related
nurse practitioners such as continence advisors, sexual counsellors and home

dialysis and diabetes specialists. Nurse practitioners will often take on a key information and advisory role, under the supervision of more senior nurses or related medical staff. In the UK there is now legislation that allows limited prescribing by qualified nurse practitioners within their own speciality area. This system does allow greater expertise to be devolved from hospitals into the community and lets people with particular disabilities access home-based advice, information and treatment more readily. A few centres are now broadening this concept with the training of therapy practitioners. The author's centre in Newcastle upon Tyne, for example, is now training a senior physiotherapist in the broad-based management of spasticity including advice on drug prescribing and the injection of botulinum toxin. A few studies have now been conducted in this field and these are reviewed in Chapter 7.

What is the role of the medical practitioner in the rehabilitation team? In the postacute hospital setting it is often the doctor who takes on the role of team leader. This may be appropriate in an acute setting, but the further away from hospital the individual progresses then the less essential the role of the doctor becomes. Obviously a properly trained consultant in rehabilitation medicine has an important role to play in any rehabilitation team. Medical training gives a broad overview of disability. The doctor has a key role to play in prescribing and advising on a whole range of treatment modalities. However, there are insufficient consultants to provide a comprehensive coverage in most countries, particularly in northern Europe. There are, for example, only about a hundred consultants in rehabilitation medicine for the whole of the UK. The background and training of such individuals normally means they are based in postacute rehabilitation units in a hospital setting. There are simply insufficient doctors to have much involvement in community teams. Ideally, at least part-time involvement of a consultant in rehabilitation medicine, or sometimes another medical discipline such as neurology, rheumatology or geriatrics, is desirable. If this is not achievable then a community rehabilitation team should have access at least to advice from a medical specialist – as it should have advice from any other 'missing' discipline. However, the absence of a medic should not discourage the formation of a rehabilitation team. The role of team leader should be the best person qualified for the task who has the appropriate leadership skills and the task should not be given by right to any particular discipline. The skills required to lead a rehabilitation team are diverse and complex and at least the individual should be able to command respect, have good communication skills, a good working knowledge of all disciplines and empathy with the fundamental principles of rehabilitation, as well as the ability to liaise with the whole range of health professionals, disabled people, managers and even politicians. The quality of charisma is also desirable! Belbin (1981) neatly summarizes the characteristics of the leader as 'someone tolerant enough to listen to others but strong enough to reject their advice'. If possible a hierarchical team structure should be avoided as this will tend to create an inflexible style of working. Burns and Stalker (1961) argued that if staff were required to find innovative solutions, as they often are in a community setting, then a hierarchically organized system can be a barrier to the production of ideas and a barrier to the appropriate sense of responsibility that may be required to establish and achieve group goals. Many writers on the subject of leadership have shown that a leader needs to be open to influence from team members. The value of listening to others is that team members may adopt decisions as their own and be more committed to achieving that particular set of goals (Ends and Page, 1977).

Many rehabilitation teams, particularly in a more diverse and geographically spread community setting, have difficulties in establishing a strong team identity. So often teams are in some form of conflict due to personality problems, role ambiguity, status difficulties or lack of any clear leadership. Teams need time to develop as teams. The 'away day' concept is valuable in developing team spirit, a common setting of principles and agreed team goals and priorities. Time to develop the rehabilitation team is essential.

Effectiveness of rehabilitation

The main purpose of this book is not to provide a complete resumé of the evidence that supports the effectiveness of rehabilitation. Obviously the purpose of this book is to review such evidence in the context of community rehabilitation. However, it is appropriate to briefly review the evidence of the effectiveness of rehabilitation as a whole. There is now considerable evidence that underpins the effectiveness of the multidisciplinary team. It is not appropriate to write a definitive review of this subject but a brief synopsis of the evidence will be given. The interested reader is referred to the supplement to the journal *Clinical Rehabilitation*, which was commissioned by the British Society of Rehabilitation Medicine and published in 1999 (BSRM, 1999).

Stroke rehabilitation

The key article in this field was the meta-analysis of stroke unit trials produced by Langhorne and colleagues in 1993 (Langhorne et al., 1993). The analysis showed about a 33% reduction in the chances of death or institutionalization at 1 year in stroke units compared with individuals managed on general medical wards. This was an influential paper and indeed has probably been one of the main driving forces leading to the more widespread establishment of stroke units in many district general hospitals in the UK and further afield. This work was largely confirmed in another meta-analysis produced by Ottenbacher and Janelle (1993). This paper reviewed a variety of studies which had used some form of functional outcome measure. The result of this meta-analysis was that, on average, individuals receiving stroke rehabilitation performed better than around two-thirds of people in the comparator groups. Finally, Kwakkel and colleagues (1997) systematically reviewed nine controlled studies with just over 1000 people after stroke in order to assess the effects of intense rehabilitation. There was a significant improvement in functional outcome in the groups with more intensive therapy. However, it is fair to point out that there were a number of criticisms of most of the controlled trials, but nevertheless this review confirmed the general trend found in the other studies and reiterated the efficacy of rehabilitation therapy after stroke. The advantage of meta-analysis and systematic review is that the deficiencies in individual studies tend to be minimized. It is not appropriate to review all individual studies that were part of the larger meta-analyses. However, one original study was influential in that it emphasized the need for continuing follow-up after initial therapy within a stroke unit. Garraway and colleagues (1980*a*) produced one of the early papers, which demonstrated the efficacy of early stroke rehabilitation. However, the follow-up study at 1 year showed that the initial benefit from early stroke rehabilitation was not sustained (Garraway et al., 1980*b*). The authors felt that lack of continued rehabilitation may have been responsible for this fall-off in initial functional gain. They also emphasized that some people may have lost some function that they gained earlier through overprotection by carers. Whatever the actual reason the study was useful in emphasizing the need for ongoing rehabilitation, follow-up and community support in order to maintain any short-term gains within the home setting. There have been a number of other studies demonstrating the efficacy of stroke rehabilitation within the community and these studies are the subject of Chapter 7.

Traumatic brain injury

There is a significant lack of good quality literature with regard to traumatic brain injury compared with the stroke literature. There is certainly no equivalent meta-analysis and indeed few studies that could be subject to such analysis. Nevertheless there are a few studies that indicate that traumatic brain injury rehabilitation may be just as efficacious as postacute stroke rehabilitation. One of the early studies often quoted is the work by Cope and Hall published in 1982. The authors compared two groups admitted early (within 35 days of injury) and late (more than 35 days postinjury). The individuals were matched for age, length of coma, disability and neurosurgical procedures. They found that disability ratings did not differ on admission, discharge or follow-up but did find that the later admission group needed twice the length of stay as the early group in order to achieve the same outcomes. A later study by the same authors (Cope et al., 1991) followed 145 people between 6 months and 2 years postinjury. Individuals were placed through a rehabilitation programme and, presumably as a result of such programme, the number of people in residential care fell from around half to 15%. The numbers engaged in productive activity increased from 6% to 35% and the number of care hours required for the group decreased from around 10 hours a day to around 4 hours a day. There were a number of criticisms of this study, including a rather inadequate outcome scale, but nevertheless the study appeared to show that holistic traumatic brain injury rehabilitation, even at later stages, seemed to be able to produce some benefit. The efficacy of later stage rehabilitation was also confirmed in the study by Tuel and colleagues (1992). In this study 49 people after traumatic brain injury were readmitted for rehabilitation at least a year postinjury. In other words these individuals were at a time when they would not be expected to make much more significant recovery. However, despite this later-stage rehabilitation the Barthel Index increased in over half the individuals. A third of them moved from dependence to assisted independence.

The intensity of therapy has also been investigated. Blackerby (1990) investigated the effects of intensive therapy. She found the length of stay was reduced by 31% when the hours of therapy were increased from 5 hours per day to 8 hours per day 7 days a week. More recent randomized trials have also shown that individuals receiving extra therapy made greater gains in independence and made such gains more rapidly (Shiel et al., 1999; Slade et al., 1999). In the latter study the group receiving enhanced therapy had a saving equivalent to 17 days in hospital.

In the specific area of behaviour modification in individuals with behavioural disturbance, Eames and Wood (1985) produced definitive work in the mid 1980s. Their unit accepted individuals at least 1 year after injury. Such people had significant behavioural problems and an intensive behavioural modification regime produced significant gains both in quality of life and in residential placement for these people.

The only study that has attempted to undertake a properly randomized assessment of traumatic brain-injury rehabilitation was published in 1998 (Semlyen et al., 1998). The authors worked in a regional inpatient rehabilitation unit. They assessed matched individuals with traumatic brain injury and compared those who went through the regional rehabilitation centre with those who were discharged from the neurosurgical unit to a nonrehabilitation environment in a local hospital or those who were discharged straight back home. The individuals were not strictly randomized. The number of inpatient beds was limited on the unit, which did not allow the unit to take all referrals and the groups were reasonably comparable. Individuals who went through the inpatient rehabilitation unit improved somewhat quicker than the comparator group and such benefits seemed to be generalizable into the community setting, given that the rehabilitation group continued to improve after discharge whereas the comparator group did not. Interestingly the degree of carer stress, as measured by the General Health Questionnaire, increased over time in the comparator group whereas it decreased over time (to a statistically significant extent at 12 months) in the rehabilitation group. This may mean that the information, support and guidance offered to carers is more effective within a rehabilitation unit, which has the desirable effect of reducing carer stress both in the short and long-term. This is a relatively unexplored area in rehabilitation and certainly worthy of further confirmatory studies.

Multiple sclerosis

Individuals with deteriorating conditions, such as multiple sclerosis, are often thought to be unlikely candidates to benefit from multidisciplinary rehabilitation. It is accepted that some drug interventions can modify the course of the disease, particularly recent studies with interferon and copolymer 1. However, the efficacy of input from a rehabilitation team is more difficult to show with any degree of robustness. Pioneering work at the National Hospital for Neurology and Neurosurgery in London has begun to demonstrate the efficacy of inpatient multidisciplinary rehabilitation for this group. Kidd and colleagues (1995) used a group of people with multiple sclerosis in the progressive stage of the disease and they acted as their own controls in a multiple single-case study design. The team assessed 79 people with multiple sclerosis and a goal-orientated management strategy was formulated. Sixty-five per cent of the people made functional gains as measured by the Barthel Index at the end of the rehabilitation period. The duration of such improvement and whether improvements in an inpatient setting can be carried over into a home environment have yet to be demonstrated. The same unit produced further work in 1996 (Freeman et al., 1996). This group reported on a waiting-list stratified randomized controlled trial. Fifty people in the progressive phase of multiple sclerosis, with a mean duration of disease of over 15 years, were randomly allocated to receive inpatient rehabilitation from the multidisciplinary team either immediately or after a 6-week waiting period. The two groups were reassessed at 6 weeks and there was significant benefit for those who had received the immediate treatment both in terms of disability and handicap, at least as measured on the Functional Independence Measure (FIM) and the London Handicap Scale. It is generally accepted that rehabilitation in multiple sclerosis is best performed in the context of the home environment. However, there are very little data that compare rehabilitation in an inpatient setting with an outpatient or community setting. One of the few studies to address this issue was produced in 1988 by Francabandera and colleagues. This group compared 67 people with chronic progressive multiple sclerosis who were randomly allocated to either inpatient or outpatient rehabilitation. The average length of stay in hospital was 3 weeks, with a similar period of outpatient rehabilitation. Assessments were performed at 3-monthly intervals and the Incapacity Status Scale was used as the outcome measure as well as the number of hours of care assistance required. Inpatient rehabilitation was found to have initial advantage over outpatient rehabilitation but such advantage was shortlived. At 1 year both groups were very similar in terms of their functional scores. The authors suggested that individuals with chronic progressive multiple sclerosis required periodic courses of rehabilitation in order to preserve small functional gains that may be achieved during each course of the rehabilitation.

Overall, the evidence in multiple sclerosis is certainly still in need of more refinement with more studies involving a larger number of people in a variety of different settings. However, the initial studies are encouraging and at least show a trend towards improvement following the application of multidisciplinary rehabilitation.

This section has briefly referred to the literature on the overall effectiveness of rehabilitation regardless of whether it is delivered in an inpatient, outpatient or community setting. The literature is far from adequate but nevertheless does demonstrate a very clear benefit from rehabilitation in the context of stroke and at least trends for benefit in the context of traumatic brain injury and multiple sclerosis. However, in the context of this book most of the definitive studies have been conducted in an inpatient and/or postacute setting. While many of these studies are encouraging it does seem likely that unless such postacute and/or inpatient rehabilitation is followed up in some way by further periods of rehabilitation either at home or in hospital, then the initial benefit seems to fade. If, in the context of this book, we can draw any conclusions from the literature then such conclusion is that community rehabilitation should be seen as an integral part of inpatient rehabilitation. The benefits of the latter may fade unless the former is also provided.

The need for community rehabilitation

The whole context of this book is to promote the need for community rehabilitation and assess the evidence for its efficacy. The case for working in the community is made both earlier in this chapter and will be developed further in other chapters. However, it may be useful at this point to summarize some of the key drivers that are moving rehabilitation towards the community.

Later problems of disability

It is well known in the literature that many of the longer-term problems associated with disability come after discharge from hospital. This is particularly applicable to individuals with acute-onset disabilities, such as stroke and traumatic brain injury. The family, for example, often have problems in adjusting to the 'personality' changes in the disabled person, after traumatic brain injury. Characteristic changes include egocentricity, childishness, poor judgement, lack of initiation, reduced drive, lethargy, disinterest, lack of depth of feeling, irritability, aggressiveness, reduced tact and an increase or decrease in sexual interest (Oddy et al., 1985; Brooks et al., 1987*a*; Karlovits and McColl, 1999). This plethora of problems will not uncommonly lead to marital disharmony or divorce as well as social isolation, alienation from previous friends and relatives and difficulties with employment. These problems may not have been particularly apparent in the early stages while the individual was in hospital. There is a tendency to focus on physical disability in the early stages and carers, and even rehabilitation teams, may give insufficient emphasis to the later-stage cognitive, intellectual, emotional and behavioural problems. When these problems emerge in the home setting then the expertise of a rehabilitation team is often required at a stage when such support may well have been withdrawn. While the disabled individual may not have much insight into their psychological problems there are often significant strains on the family. However, often the individual is aware of such difficulties and there is increasing anxiety and depression in the months and years after the acute event. Once again such difficulties will often occur when the individual is back in the community after hospital support has been withdrawn. Longer-term difficulties not only affect family and social relationships but also have impact on employment. There is no doubt that the employment rate is significantly lower in disabled people in general but in particular in those with neurological problems. Brooks and colleagues (1987*b*) followed up 98 people with severe head injuries between 2 and 7 years after injury. In this group employment rate fell from 86% preinjury to just 29% postinjury. A number of other studies have confirmed the low rate of return to work after acute neurological events and in longer-term deteriorating neurological conditions.

Overall the literature is clear that there is a significant range of problems that occur in the months and years after initial neurological insult. Provision of a postacute rehabilitation facility only serves the needs of people with neurological disabilities for a short part of their lifespan with a disability. It is illogical not to provide longer-term community rehabilitation.

The views of disabled people

Chapter 5 summarizes the views of disabled people, particularly within the context of the social model of disability. The reader is referred to that chapter but in summary it is very clear that people with disabilities both need and require longer-term support services to be based within the home setting or at least within the local community. As commissioners of healthcare take more notice of the views of customers then it is also right that much more account be taken of such views when planning health services. This is another significant driver at redirecting health resources into the community.

Increasing autonomy of nonmedical health practitioners

There are increasing numbers of health professionals working in the community. For many years general practitioners/family physicians have been supported by a range of professionals, particularly nurses. In the UK the nursing subprofessions of district nursing and health visiting are well established. Naturally such individuals have always been involved from a health perspective with disabled people living at home. However, in recent years we have seen the growth of the specialist nurse. These individuals are usually trained in specific subjects, such as multiple sclerosis, Parkinson's disease, epilepsy, etc. The initial trend was for such appointments to be supported by pharmaceutical companies, although many individuals are now within the mainstream health service. The training is generally rather ad hoc. Some individuals are attached to local neurology departments and work on an outreach basis while others are purely community based. However, there is a clear trend for such individuals to work within the community in a specialist setting with people with particular disabilities. The UK government has supported this development and indeed given such individuals increasing autonomy with regard to prescribing within fixed protocols. They are, effectively, junior doctors working in a single subject area. The growth of nurse practitioners has been somewhat haphazard and the training and quality standards have not been subject to rigorous scrutiny. This situation is changing as the UK nursing hierarchy begins to formulate appropriate training programmes and monitor quality standards. In addition to nursing developments there are now more therapists working purely in a community setting. Once again such individuals have always been available in small numbers in the community. Physiotherapy, occupational therapy and chiropody have had a long history of community working. Occupational therapists, for example, have for many years been employed by local social service departments in the UK and have played a key role in aids and adaptations for disabled people living within their homes. Community therapists have begun to grow in number and around the country groups of therapists, and nurses, have begun to coalesce into community-based rehabilitation teams. There are many models of working, sometimes from outreach hospital bases or sometimes working entirely in the community. Some teams are totally employed by the NHS while others are largely employees of local social service departments. There are some teams in the private sector who may have an increased focus on vocational rehabilitation or community reintegration. Such teams often attract funding from the medicolegal system. Some teams have a diagnostic focus and concentrate, for example, exclusively on people with multiple sclerosis or epilepsy. Other teams are more generically based physical disability teams while others have different age limits. The growth of community rehabilitation teams has certainly been patchy and many parts of the UK are without any such support.

The reality is that health systems have seen a steady growth of community rehabilitation in the context of nonmedical health professionals. There is very limited medical involvement in most teams although there are some notable exceptions. There are now a few community-orientated geriatricians, paediatricians or rehabilitation physicians working, at least part-time, in the community. This increasing independence and autonomy from the medical hierarchy is a further key driver for the development of community teams. Other European countries have seen similar growth but, in general, such growth has been patchier, particularly in southern Europe. The concept of nonmedical health professional teams in many countries is still alien to the local culture.

Developments in the health service

There has been a radical change in health politics in recent years. In the UK there has been a clear shift of emphasis from acute hospitals to the community. The majority of health commissioning in the UK is now through Primary Care Trusts. These are semi-autonomous bodies within the umbrella of the UK NHS. The Trusts have a responsibility for commissioning health service in their locality both in the community and in hospital. The board of such Trusts has a predominance of community practitioners, particularly general practitioners. Naturally this change has resulted in more commissioning resources being placed within the community and less towards acute hospitals. Many hospitals, particularly in larger cities, have seen a significant reduction in bed numbers with a consequent need to develop innovative ideas both to keep people out of hospital and to discharge them quicker once they have been admitted. This has led to the growth, albeit uncoordinated, of various models of outreach teams and early-discharge teams. Some theoretical models are described below and other specific models are described in later chapters. The trend to move resources from institutional hospitals into the community is one that is seen across many developed parts of the world.

Thus, there are four main drivers that are moving services towards the community. First, the clear, evidence-based realization that most problems associated with neurological disability occur when the individual is back at home. These problems are often associated with community and social reintegration and re-employment. Second, there is the clear view of disabled people and their lobby organizations that more resources should be placed within the community for longer-term support. Third, there is the trend towards increasing autonomy of therapists and nurses who are also becoming more prevalent in a community setting. Finally, there is the government-backed change in the health service, which is also placing more emphasis on commissioning and provision of services within localities. Thus, there is a clear need for serious consideration to be given to neurological rehabilitation services to be much more focused in the community while, of course, being careful not to strip resources away from the excellent network of postacute rehabilitation, hospital-based units.

Theoretical models

This section outlines some of the theoretical models that might underpin a community rehabilitation programme. Specific examples are obviously annotated throughout this book and in particular in the evidence-based review in Chapter 7. Thus, this section will not attempt to describe actual examples but describe the theoretical possibilities and outline some of the advantages and disadvantages of such possibilities.

Whatever model of service delivery is adopted each rehabilitation team should have a basic set of principles which underpin their work. Clearly each team must adopt principles according to its own particular circumstances. However, a reasonable starting point may be the key principles for the involvement of disabled people as outlined by the Prince of Wales Advisory Group on Disability (1985). These principles, adjusted for adoption by a rehabilitation team, are as follows:

Choice – the team should aim to provide disabled people with a choice regarding where they live and how they maintain their independence, including help in learning how to choose.

Consultation – every team should consult widely with disabled people and their families on services as they are planned and developed.

Information – should be clearly presented and readily available to all disabled consumers who may access the team.

Participation – the team should promote the participation of disabled people in the life of the local community as far as possible.

Recognition – the team should recognize that long-term disability is not synonymous with illness and that the medical model of care is inappropriate in the majority of cases.

Autonomy – the team should enable disabled people to make their own decisions regarding a way of life best suited to their own personal circumstances.

It may be useful to add to this published list a few other basic principles pertinent to the delivery of healthcare within a community environment.

Clinical access – a person with a neurological disability should be able to access information, advice and treatment from an appropriate clinical expert. Such expertise should, as far as possible, be without undue delay within an accessible environment and within a reasonable geographical distance of the individual's home.

If the team adheres to these basic principles then the team structure and mode of delivery becomes less relevant.

Hospital outpatients

If the basis of most rehabilitation is the hospital-based rehabilitation department then a step towards the community could involve the establishment of outpatient follow-up systems based within the same hospital/rehabilitation centre. This is probably the most prevalent model as the majority of hospital units almost certainly have some form of outpatient follow-up system. As we have stated in this book, and will state again in subsequent chapters, long-term support is vital in order to maintain the short-term benefits that may have accrued from time in a rehabilitation unit. In theory an outpatient support system is able to offer such support. Individuals can be monitored and further periods of rehabilitation delivered as necessary. The outpatient department can serve as a source of advice and information. In some circumstances the outpatient department can act as a social centre for gathering of people with similar disabilities or diagnoses. This may encourage the formation of self-help groups that are also based within the same environment. In logistical terms such arrangements can make sense as the same rehabilitation team can work from the same building, thus providing both continuity of care and preventing the need for potentially long periods of time away from base. Significant numbers of people can be seen in a single outpatient clinic compared with the travel of team members to individual's homes. A clinic for the injection of botulinum toxin, invaluable for the management of dystonia and spasticity, is an example where it is likely that necessary expertise would only be available in one or a few localities. However, it is obvious that while there are some advantages to such a system, given limited resources, an outpatient department fails to fulfil basic requirements of community rehabilitation. It has to be accepted that in many circumstances such a model is unavoidable, particularly if there is such limited expertise that the few experts simply do not have the time to travel around the local community.

Disease-specific clinics

An adaptation of the outpatient system is the use of disease- or symptom-based clinics. Examples would be clinics for people with multiple sclerosis or Parkinson's disease or clinics specifically for those with continence problems or spasticity. The same advantages apply as with generic outpatient departments. Perhaps an additional advantage is the more readily available social and peer support that may come from associated groups, such as the Multiple Sclerosis Society or the Dystonia Society, etc. Such a system may be relevant to some groups but there are clearly logistic problems about establishing a suitable range of clinics to suit all different diseases and relevant symptoms. It is more than likely that many rarer symptoms and diseases would simply

have no appropriate support. Obviously the essentials of community rehabilitation would still not apply to this model.

Hospital outreach teams

A logical extension of the hospital-based multidisciplinary rehabilitation
team is for that team to additionally work in the community. Individual team
members could continue to work with the same disabled person whether they
are in hospital or in the community and this would have some advantage
with regard to continuity of management. The team would be able to provide longer-term support and ongoing rehabilitation. However, increased
resources would be a prerequisite to enable sufficient team members to be
employed in the same team and thus allow appropriate coverage of the geographical area. It is likely that the hospital unit would serve a considerable
geographical region, which the outreach team would need to cover. It is also
likely that considerable time would be lost in travelling and one can see logistical problems of organizing appropriate team members to be in the right
place at the right time. However, such teams have been successful, particularly in the context of early discharge from hospital following, for example,
a stroke (see Chapter 7). The numbers of disabled people will obviously
slowly increase over time and one can also foresee circumstances in which
the outreach team would begin to be overwhelmed by numbers over a large
geographical area.

Extension of primary care teams

In the UK a potential base for community rehabilitation is attachment to the
general practitioner and primary care team. A typical group general practice
has a population of around 10 000. Thus, the numbers of disabled people are
reduced to a more practical level. Contact would be maintained with basic
healthcare services and referral could be made to the local hospital rehabilitation department as required. However, there are two clear disadvantages
to attaching a community rehabilitation team to a general practice. First,
many diseases and disabilities are relatively rare. A general practitioner, for
example, is likely to see only one new person with multiple sclerosis once
every 20 years. Even commoner conditions, such as stroke, may be seen by a
general practitioner only three or four times a year. This reduces the level of
expertise and experience. If the primary care team is general practitioner-led

then its lack of experience coupled with the varying interests in physical disability may lead to a patchy and uncoordinated service to the community as a whole. In addition many experts, particularly in the therapy professions, are few and far between and it is most unlikely that the necessary expertise would be found to adequately support each primary care team. Thus, it seems that a larger geographical base is required than a primary care team but a smaller geographical base than the typical hospital catchment area.

Primary care team support

In view of the comments above, a compromise model is for the primary healthcare team to be supported by occasional visits by members of the specialist rehabilitation team. Such a project was designed in Southampton in the south of the UK with the support of the Parkinson's Disease Society. In this particular project a consultant in neurological rehabilitation attended meetings with the primary care teams in four different group general practices for discussion of specific people with Parkinson's disease. The consultant, without seeing the individual, was able to make a range of recommendations and offer practical advice and support to the general practitioners. Such a model could be envisaged with other members of the rehabilitation team with, for example, specialist nurses advising the district nurse attached to the practice of the general practitioner.

Community-based teams

A logical extension of the above argument is for an expert multidisciplinary rehabilitation team to be based in the community but covering a geographical area that is sensible both in terms of numbers of disabled people and geographical spread. A population base of around 100 000 may provide appropriate numbers. However, this number is no more than a general guideline as clearly the actual number will depend on local resources and circumstances, local geography and, of course, appropriate availability of the necessary expert team members. A problem with a community-based team is, at least theoretically, professional isolation. The team would need to liaise with other teams or with the local hospital centre or regional rehabilitation centre. Such links would be necessary for referral of particularly complex difficulties as well as for audit, education and training. An example, known to the authors, is the Newcastle community multiple sclerosis team. This is a self-contained expert multidisciplinary team, led by a physiotherapist. It is based in a local disabled living centre but the majority of work is conducted within individual's homes. The team has managerial and professional links with the Newcastle-based regional rehabilitation centre. The team is able to access beds within that centre for emergency or respite purposes or for periods of rehabilitation after, for example, a relapse. This model is often referred to as 'hub and spoke'. In a broad geographical area a number of such teams could interlink, sharing educational opportunities, staff training and being joint employers of particular experts who could spend some time in a number of individual teams. This concept is sometimes termed a managed clinical network.

Health-based or social service-based?

In the UK and many European countries there is a clear distinction between health services, which are often nationally organized, and social services, which are often locally organized. The former provides healthcare whereas the latter provides a variety of social support including personal assistance at home, home cleaning and shopping support, benefits advice and locally organized aids and adaptations within the home. The local government would run the social services department as well as the housing department, which would provide local rented housing. As individuals move away from hospital the need for continuing health input becomes less while at the same time the need for social service input usually increases. Thus, it is somewhat artificial to provide a community-based health team in isolation from the local social service department. Ideally such a team should have individuals from both camps in order to provide a single rehabilitation service in a given locality. Preferably such teams would also share budgets to save endless budgetary disputes. A local example, known to the authors, is the Northumberland Head Injury Service. This team has an administrative base in a small hospital and shares this facility with the local Headway group – a branch of the national society for people with traumatic brain injury. The team has members both from the health service and the local social services and is led by a health-employed social worker. The team has close educational and professional links with the regional rehabilitation centre in Newcastle as well as the local neurosurgical unit. The team is able to see every individual with a head injury in the county of Northumberland and will usually see such people in their own home and follow them up for as long as is required. They have access to both health and social service budgets and thus can directly access both NHS and social service facilities.

Such broad-based teams should help to promote fuller participation of the disabled person in the local community.

Ideally, such teams should not be restricted to just the health and social services but should also involve other relevant professionals. This could include, for example, access to employment rehabilitation advice (Department of Employment), advice on disability benefits (Department of Social Security) and a whole range of other professionals and services, such as medicolegal experts and voluntary organizations.

Independent Living Movement

If the aim of the community rehabilitation team is to empower local disabled people then it is logical that at least some disabled people should be able to organize their own rehabilitation services. Collective groups of disabled people or even individual disabled people could be enabled to request assistance from an appropriate range of professionals as and when needed. There are some examples in the UK of local authorities giving disabled people their own budget to buy such services as required. This model is firmly supported by the Independent Living Movement and by disabled person's groups, such as the British Council of Organizations for Disabled People (Brisenden, 1986). This might be an ideal solution for certain groups of disabled people, particularly those who are cognitively intact, but becomes rather less satisfactory when dealing with people with cognitive and intellectual problems. There are some disabled people who simply could not manage their own affairs. An appropriately trained advocate or an appropriate family member could support such people. Obviously such a model would require access to a broad range of relevant and understandable information otherwise people may not access appropriate individuals at the appropriate times.

Resource centres – towards an ideal model?

One model that is emerging in some parts of the UK and Europe is the community resource centre. These centres are local and fully accessible, particularly in terms of public transport. Resource centres should provide a reliable information service and often provide an administrative base for local self-help groups. Such centres can be run by groups of disabled people with or without professional support. The centres could be the base for the local community rehabilitation team or could even act as an appropriate outstation for the local hospital or regional rehabilitation centre. Ideally, the centres could also act as a base for social and recreational activities as well as other relevant services such as vocational training, counselling and social functions. Preferably, such resource centres should not be viewed as facilities only for disabled people but could well be used by the local community for other community groups and services. A centre along these lines has recently been established in Liverpool in the UK with a grant from a multinational pharmaceutical company.

These are some theoretical examples of models of service delivery within a community setting. There are certainly many other permutations. Some further examples are given in later chapters. There is no single model that should be imposed. Each community needs to look at its present facilities, health and social service resources and the ability to access other relevant agencies. After such a review an appropriate model will usually become apparent. The essence of community rehabilitation should be flexibility. A model of service adapted one year may not be right the following year as different circumstances may have arisen. The community team should be seen as a highly flexible concept that needs to change and adjust as it develops.

REFERENCES

Bax, M., Smythe, D. and Thomas, A. (1998). Health care of physically handicapped young adults. *British Medical Journal* **290**, 1153–5.

Belbin, R.M. (1981). *Management Teams*. London: Heinemann.

Blackerby, W.F. (1990). Intensity of rehabilitation and length of stay. *Brain Injury* **4**, 167–73.

Brisenden, S. (1986). Independent living in a medical model of disability. *Disability, Handicap and Society* **1**, 173–81.

British Society of Rehabilitation Medicine (1998). *Rehabilitation after Traumatic Brain Injury*. London: BSRM.

British Society of Rehabilitation Medicine (1999). The effectiveness of rehabilitation: a critical review of the evidence. *Clinical Rehabilitation* **13** (Suppl. 1), 1–81.

Brooks, D.N., Campsie, L., Symington, C. et al. (1987*a*). The effects of severe head injury on the patient and relative within seven years of injury. *Journal of Head Trauma Rehabilitation* **2**, 1–13.

Brooks, D.N., McKinlay, W.W., Symington, C. et al. (1987*b*). Return to work within the first seven years of severe head injury. *Brain Injury* **1**, 5–19.

Burns, T. and Stalker, G.M. (1961). *The Management of Innovation*. London: Tavistock.

Bury, M. (2000). A comment on the ICIDH II. *Disability and Society* **15**, 1073–7.

Cope, N. and Hall, K. (1982). Head injury rehabilitation: benefits of early intervention. *Archives of Physical Medicine and Rehabilitation* **63**, 433–7.

Cope, N.D., Cole, J.R., Hall, K. and Barkans, H. (1991). Brain injury: analysis of outcome in a post-acute rehabilitation system. Part I. General analysis. *Brain Injury* **5**, 111–25.

Eames, P. and Wood, R. (1985). Rehabilitation after severe brain injury: a follow-up study of a behavioural modification approach. *Journal of Neurology, Neurosurgery and Psychiatry* **48**, 613–19.

Ends, E.J. and Page, C.W. (1977). *Organizational Team Building*. Cambridge, MA: Winthrop.

Francabandera, F.L., Holland, N.J., Wiesel-Levison, P. and Scheinberg, L.C. (1988). Multiple sclerosis rehabilitation: inpatient versus outpatient. *Rehabilitation Nursing* **13**, 251–3.

Freeman, J., Langdon, D., Hobart, J. and Thompson, A.J. (1996). The impact of rehabilitation on disability and handicap in progressive multiple sclerosis: a randomized controlled trial. *European Journal of Neurology* **3** (Suppl. 2), 15.

Garraway, W.M., Akhtar, A.J., Hockey, L. and Prescott, R.J. (1980*a*). Management of acute stroke in the elderly: preliminary results of a controlled trial. *British Medical Journal* **280**, 1040–4.

Garraway, W.M., Akhtar, A.J., Hockey, L. and Prescott, R.J. (1980*b*). Management of acute stroke in the elderly: follow-up of a controlled trial. *British Medical Journal* **281**, 827–9.

Karlovits, T. and McColl, M.A. (1999) Coping with community reintegration after severe brain injury: a description of stresses and coping strategies. *Brain Injury* **13**, 845–61.

Kidd, D., Howard, R.S., Losseff, N.A. and Thompson, A.J. (1995). The benefit of inpatient neurorehabilitation in multiple sclerosis. *Clinical Rehabilitation* **9**, 198–203.

Kwakkel, G., Wagenaar, R.C., Koelman, T.W. et al. (1997). The effects of intensity of rehabilitation after stroke. A research synthesis. *Stroke* **28**, 1550–6.

Langhorne, P., Williams, B.O., Gilchrist, W. and Howie, K. (1993). Do stroke units save lives? *Lancet* **342**, 395–8.

Langton-Hewer, R. (1993). The epidemiology of disabling neurological disorders. In *Neurological rehabilitation*, ed. R. Greenwood, M. Barnes, T. McMillan and C. Ward, pp. 3–12. Edinburgh: Churchill Livingston.

Martin, J., Meltzer, H. and Elliot, D. (1988). *The Prevalence of Disability among Young Adults*. OPCS Report 1. London: HMSO.

Oddy, M., Coughlan, T., Tyerman, A. and Jenkins, D. (1985). Social adjustment after closed head injury: a further follow-up seven years after injury. *Journal of Neurology, Neurosurgery and Psychiatry* **48**, 564–8.

Ottenbacher, K.J. and Janelle, S. (1993). The results of clinical trials in stroke rehabilitation research. *Archives of Neurology* **50**, 37–44.

Oxfordshire Community Stroke Project (1983). Incidence of stroke in Oxfordshire: first years' experience of a community stroke register. *British Medical Journal* **287**, 713–17.

Pfeiffer, D. (2000). The devils are in the details: the ICIDH II and the disability movement. *Disability and Society* **15**, 1079–82.

Rosen, M.G. and Dickinson, J.C. (1992). The incidence of cerebral palsy. *American Journal of Obstetrics and Gynaecology* **167**, 417–23.

Semlyen, J.K., Summers, S.J. and Barnes, M.P. (1998). Traumatic brain injury: efficacy of multidisciplinary rehabilitation. *Archives of Physical Medicine and Rehabilitation* **79**, 678–83.

Shiel, A., Henry, D., Clark, J. et al. (1999). Effect of increased intervention on rate of functional recovery after brain injury: preliminary results of a controlled trial. *Clinical Rehabilitation* **13**, 90.

Slade, A., Chamberlain, M.A. and Tennant, A. (1999). Enhancing therapy: does it make a difference? *Clinical Rehabilitation* **13**, 94.

The Prince of Wales Advisory Group on Disability (1985). *Living Options*. London: Prince of Wales Advisory Group on Disability.

Tuel, S.M., Presty, S.K., Meythaler, J.M. et al. (1992). Functional improvement in severe head injury after re-admission for rehabilitation. *Brain Injury* **6**, 363–72.

Wade, D. and Langton-Hewer, R. (1987). Epidemiology of some neurological diseases, with specific reference to workload on the NHS. *International Rehabilitation Medicine* **8**, 129–37.

World Health Organization (1980). *International Classification of Impairments, Disabilities and Handicaps*. Albany, NY: WHO.

World Health Organization (1999). *International Classification of Functioning and Disability – Beta-2 draft*. Geneva: WHO.

3

Models of disability

Introduction

In the context of community rehabilitation it is particularly important to define the underlying philosophy of service delivery. The predominant model underlying most healthcare provision across the world is the so-called 'medical model'. However, in recent years disabled people themselves and their lobbyists have been promoting an alternative view of disability – the 'social model'. This chapter will describe the principles of each model to ensure that the reader can take on board the purpose and implications of the different approaches to disability. However, it is important to emphasize that these two models of disability are not entirely incompatible. A comprehensive health service probably needs to draw on some aspects of both models so that health professionals and disabled people can work together to ensure that high-quality rehabilitation is delivered to all those that need it in an equitable and participative fashion.

The purpose of models

Models attempt to provide a framework through which the understanding of a concept can be easily grasped. The challenge is to make sense of often complex and multifaceted concepts in simple ways. Creating models offer ways in which to make sense of the world. Ultimately, however, they are artificial constructions of ideas that are not created so as to fit neatly into rigid frameworks. Thus, probably there are no models that adequately reflect the entirety of a concept. Different models propose explanations for the same concept in different ways, but really they may only represent different components of the same concept.

Models are dynamic. They are continually adapted or recreated to better reflect what we know and understand. However, our knowledge is rarely fixed. It is shaped and influenced by beliefs, attitudes and behaviours prevalent in society at the time and consequently is ever-changing. Therefore we are faced with the prospect of using, creating and working with models that are never definitive and never quite right. Rather models serve to provide the basis from which knowledge can be nurtured. Models are fluid structures that facilitate understanding, presenting a theoretical framework from which practice can flourish. Insights from direct practical experience feed back into the model, fuelling its dynamic constitution. Ultimately, models should be recognized for what they are – vehicles for understanding. They are not an answer in themselves. If this is understood then models present an invaluable resource for continual development.

Models in the field of disability are complex because disability means different things for different people. 'Disability, like most dimensions of experience, is polysemic – that is ambiguous and unstable in meaning' (Bricher, 2000). The two models prevalent in the field of disability – medical and social – have been widely thought to be mutually incompatible. Indeed, in the early days of the disability movement, these two concepts did represent opposite ends of the spectrum of disability philosophy and there was little overlap in the models and virtually no communication between their proponents. However, if we accept that models must be flexible and reflect changes in society then they will have to readjust to incorporate new ideas and new approaches. Community rehabilitation, by definition, is moving away from the medically orientated hospital and institutional focus. Thus, as this type of health support develops it provides a good opportunity to study potential overlaps between the different models of disability and perhaps work towards greater understanding and integration.

Models are the theoretical groundwork for practical application. They present a way in which we can understand disability and relate to it. The way in which disability is perceived has enormous implications for the way in which disabled people are treated and recognized in society. Delivery of healthcare in a community setting is a fundamental part of this equation.

The medical model of disability

There is no doubt about the enormous benefits that have arisen as a direct result of medicine and medical practice, particularly in the last century. Many diseases that once caused impairments can now be largely prevented. Polio is one such example of a disease of steeply declining incidence due to advances in medical science. The disabling effects of accidents can now be ameliorated by prompt medical and surgical intervention. Few would doubt the value of a medically dominated health system at times of acute illness or serious injury. However, people with impairments are not always ill and it can be strongly argued that an illness model of disability is not appropriate. Regrettably, the medical speciality of rehabilitation has come from an 'illness' background. It is a specialism that, in general, is carried out by physicians with the support of nurses and therapists and delivered to disabled people. This health- and illness-related perspective of disability is what is known as the medical model of disability. It assumes several things about the nature of disability. These are outlined below, as based on the concepts proposed by Lang (1998).

- Disability is individualized. It is regarded as a disease state that is located within an individual. Thus, the problem and solution may both be found within that individual.
- As disability is a disease state or abnormality, a deviation from the norm, it inherently necessitates some form of treatment or cure.
- Disability can rarely be 'cured' and thus the terms 'rehabilitation' and 'rehabilitation medicine' evolve, so as to better describe the process of medical intervention that aims to normalize.
- Being disabled a person is regarded as inherently biologically or psychologically inferior to that of the able-bodied and normal human being.
- Disability is a personal tragedy. It assumes the presence of a victim.
- The objective normality state that is assumed by professionals gives them a dominant decision-making role often noted in the typical doctor/patient relationship.

The medical model itself employs 'ab-normality'. The philosophy of medicine is to treat and cure but in the case of rehabilitation, where this outcome is unlikely, the aim is rather to normalize. This philosophy was reinforced by the World Health Organization when it accepted the distinction between impairment, disability and handicap as first proposed in 1971. *The*

Table 3.1. Definitions of the *International Classification of Impairments, Disabilities and Handicaps* (WHO, 1980)

Impairment	Any loss or abnormality of psychological, physiological or anatomical structure or function
Disability	Any restriction or lack of activity resulting from an impairment to perform an activity in the manner or in the range considered normal for people of the same age, sex and culture
Handicap	A disadvantage for a given individual resulting from impairment or disability that limits or prevents the fulfilment of a role that would otherwise be normal for that individual

International Classification of Impairment, Disability and Handicap (ICIDH) was originally published in 1980 (WHO, 1980). In a sense the ICIDH classification was a step forward from a very narrow medical model of health and disease, which was primarily concerned with body systems and diagnoses. At least the new classification recognized the consequences of health-related phenomena. The classification did recognize the problems of social disadvantage – 'handicap' – but nevertheless the classification was still rooted in a medical model with emphasis still placed on abnormality, disability and disadvantage. The actual definitions used in the ICIDH are shown in Table 3.1.

The ICIDH has widely underpinned the development of rehabilitation medicine in most countries. It has been used in many ways, from population surveys of disabilities (Martin et al., 1988) to more applied healthcare settings (e.g. the development of the London Handicap Scale; Harwood et al., 1994) and sociological research. However, while the ICIDH was an advance for its time and has provided a useful framework to underpin the introduction of rehabilitation in modern health systems it is nevertheless still surrounded with controversy. The ICIDH makes clear links between health-related disorders, chronic illness and disablement, which is an anathema to many disabled people and the disability movement in general. This is somewhat ironic as the intention of the ICIDH was to put social exclusion on the healthcare agenda (Bury, 2000).

In addition to the confined definitions of the ICIDH, rehabilitation has tended to have firm roots in a hospital- and institutional-based system. Most rehabilitation across the world, if it exists at all, exists on hospital wards, hospital-based rehabilitation units and occasionally separate but still institutional rehabilitation centres. Long-term provision for those with severe impairments who cannot live at home or in the community have historically been provided in hospital-like institutions (e.g. Leonard Cheshire Homes in the UK). This institutional focus has simply reinforced the medical model. Healthcare purchasers have further reinforced the normalization process by generally funding only short-term postacute rehabilitation following personal catastrophes such as stroke and traumatic brain injury. Health funding for longer-term support and community rehabilitation provision has been singularly lacking. Rehabilitation in the later years of the twentieth century was thus characterized by rehabilitation in a hospital or institutional setting delivered *by* the medical profession, with the support of nursing and therapy professionals, *to* disabled people. In this context it is perhaps not surprising that there has arisen a substantial challenge to this medical perspective of disability. This challenge is commonly known as the social model of disability.

The social model of disability

Disability is something imposed on top of our impairments by the way we are unnecessarily isolated and excluded from full participation in society. (UPIAS, 1976)

In order to recognize the language and conceptual problems associated with the ICIDH the World Health Organization has recently adopted a new classification (Table 3.2). This is known as the Beta II version or the ICIDH2. In this version the term 'disability' has been replaced by 'activity' and the term 'handicap' has been replaced by 'participation'. The changes are more detailed but this is the essence of the new version. This undoubtedly places a more positive spin on disability with clearly more emphasis on activity and participation in society rather than alienation from it. However, this version is still criticized by the disability movement (Pfeiffer, 2000). The disability movement still feels that the underlying paradigm of both the ICIDH and ICIDH2 is the sick role and the reinforcement of medical dominance. It is felt that the classification still medicalizes disability, places emphasis on normality and stresses causality between impairment which in turn causes disability which in turn causes disadvantage. The classification system also paves the way for the government to put a price on quality of life in the form of benefits.

Table 3.2. New classification of the *International Classification of Functioning and Disability – ICIDH2*

Impairment	The loss or abnormality of body structure of a physiological or psychological function
Activity	The nature and extent of functioning at the level of the person. Activities may be limited in nature, duration and quality
Contextual factors	Include the features, aspects and attributes of objects, structures, human-made organizations, service provision and agencies in the physical, social and attitudinal environment in which people live and conduct their lives. Contextual factors include both environmental factors and personal factors

Source: Halbertsma et al., 2000.

There is no doubting some of the principles underlying the social model. It is clearly too simplistic to imply that impairment in itself is the sole cause of social disadvantage. There are obviously other factors that come into play including the attitude of society, physical barriers and significant difficulties with poverty and unemployment. If this is the case why is the social model not more accepted? There are a number of possible reasons. It may be that the model is not widely known and understood. It may be that it has become associated with a rather extreme and anti-establishment view of life. It may be that it threatens the status quo and potentially undermines the status of medical and other health professionals. It may also be that the model itself does not provide a practical and immediate solution to the real day-to-day difficulties experienced by disabled people. It is a conceptual model and not an immediately achievable practical model. It is also worth bearing in mind that many people in receipt of rehabilitation services do not identify with being disabled. Their concept of themselves does not include the disabled identity and their thoughts about rehabilitation are likely to be focused on cure, or at least the ability to approach normality as closely as possible. Some individuals, for example, with spinal cord injury strive, by whatever means, to stand on their two feet even if such ambulation is inefficient and clumsy compared with wheelchair use.

The fundamental construct behind the social model of disability is that a person's impairment is not the cause of the restriction of activity which is imposed on people who are labelled disabled. It is the organization of society that discriminates against them and presumes that people labelled disabled can do little or nothing of value. In the view of many disabled people in the disability movement there are many barriers that prevent full integration into society. Attitudinal, sensory, architectural and economic barriers are equally, if not more, important than health barriers. The social model focuses on the opinion that disability is a construction of society. If society could accept and accommodate disabled people both physically and attitudinally then disability as a concept would be made redundant. The social model reacts against disability being viewed primarily in a negative way. *Collins Dictionary and Thesaurus* summarizes the negative connotations surrounding disability – 'affliction, ailment, complaint, defect, disablement, disorder, handicap, impairment, infirmity, malady, disqualification, impotency, inability, incapacity, incompetency, unfitness, weakness'. Disability is laden with negative connotations. The word 'disability' in itself implies a lack, a deprivation of some sort. It places value on the whole. It is a concept constructed by society – the ideal image being a fully functioning individual and anything that deviates from this norm being considered unhealthy or inferior. Disabled people tend to be viewed in the light of their disabilities as opposed to their abilities (Brisenden, 1986). A polarized view of the social model of disability implies rejection of the involvement of health professionals in the life of the person with the disability. The medical role is accepted if the disabled person happens to be ill but a role in the assistance or management of the disability itself is rejected. In this model cooperation between disabled people, their families and the medical and health professions is difficult. It is hard to see how anyone benefits from a mutually antagonistic position. Is there a middle ground?

A model for community rehabilitation

The 'strong' social model necessitates that change should occur within the social environment and not within the individual. However, there is a danger of overstating the role of the social organization and ignoring the reality of the body (Imrie, 1997). As Shakespeare and Watson (2002) state ' . . . there is no reason why appropriate action on impairment – and even various forms of impairment prevention – cannot coexist with action to remove disabling environments and practices. People are disabled both by social barriers and by their bodies'. As described earlier, models need to be dynamic and adaptable in order to keep up with current trends. It is probable that we need to leave the medical and social models on the back burner and progress to the next generation of models. In the words of Shakespeare and Erickson (2000) 'we believe that an adequate social theory of disability would include all dimensions of disabled peoples' experiences: bodily, psychological, cultural, social, political, rather than claiming that disability is either medical or social'.

As rehabilitation services develop in the community there is a need to readdress the polarized models of disability and explore the middle ground. It can be viewed that the two models are at opposite ends of a continuum and a potential for interaction is limited. Many advocates of the social model would deny there is a possibility for any integration between the two models because they are based on entirely different constructs. Indeed the social model arose in direct opposition to and in face of the dominance of the medical model. However, if rehabilitation services are to progress and develop then middle ground should be explored. Community rehabilitation will tend to work with people with longer-term impairments and the social implications of those problems will be more apparent than in an institutional and more postacute setting. There is a need to work with other agencies such as the education, employment, social service, voluntary and leisure sectors. There is a more pressing requirement for impairments to be looked at in a societal context than purely from a medical and health viewpoint. There is more need for professionals working in the field to recognize, understand and empathize with the concepts lying behind the social model. Are there practical steps that can be taken to mould these models into a more coherent whole?

First, health professionals working in the community should strive to understand the concepts lying behind the social model of disability and receive compulsory disability awareness training. Such knowledge should assist individuals to move away from a narrower health and illness orientation. Second, if disability groups exist within the community setting then contact should be made and dialogue started. If, as is regrettably common, no disability groups or societies meet in the locality then health professionals could usefully try to stimulate such groups to come into being. The voice of the individual disabled person is important but the collective voice of disabled people is usually louder. Third, once dialogue has started between the disability community and health professionals then this dialogue should be used to design the service requirements. This should allow the views of disabled people to have a real influence on the establishment of locally orientated services. Fourth, once services are established then disabled people and disability groups should be involved in continuing to monitor and develop the service. Ideally, if local politics allow, disabled people should carry responsibility for the service hand-in-hand with the professionals.

Lessons from the South (see Chapter 8) usually indicate that community rehabilitation services are only successful if they are designed and supported by disabled people. The nature of rehabilitation services is that they are health related but this should not stop these services being designed, supported, maintained and monitored by the local disabled community. Furthermore, when the diversity of the concept of disability is embraced it may create the bedrock from which partnership can grow.

This chapter has described the concepts that lie behind the two traditional models prevalent in the field of disability and rehabilitation – the medical model and the social model. It is important for practitioners to understand the philosophy that lies behind these two models but at the same time adopting a polarized view is inappropriate in a community-based service. Community services, more so than hospital services, need to work closely not only with the disabled person and their family but also with the local community and the local disabled community. Professionals working in this field strive towards a partnership with the community of disabled people. It is not to deny their own skills and professional backgrounds but is simply to recognize support and nurture the positive contribution that disabled people can and should make in a modern multicultural society.

REFERENCES

Bricher, G. (2000). Disabled people, health professionals and the social model of disability: can there be a research relationship? *Disability and Society* **15**, 781–93.

Brisenden, S. (1986). Independent living and the medical model. *Disability, Handicap and Society* **1**, 173–8.

Bury, M. (2000). A comment on the ICIDH 2. *Disability and Society* **15**, 1073–7.

Halbertsma, J., Heerkens, Y.F., Hirs, W.M. et al. (2000). Towards a new ICIDH. International classification of impairments, disabilities and handicaps. *Disability and Rehabilitation* **22**, 144–56.

Harwood, R.H., Rogers, A., Dickinson, E. and Ebrahim, S. (1994). Measuring handicap: the London Handicap Scale. A new outcome measure for chronic disease. *Quality in Health Care* **3**, 11–16.

Imrie, R. (1997). Rethinking the relationships between disability, rehabilitation and society. *Disability and Rehabilitation* **19**, 263–71.

Martin, J., Meltzer, H. and Elliot, D. (1988). *The Prevalence of Disability among Adults*. OPCS Report 1. London: HMSO.

Lang, R. (1998). A critique of the Disability Movement. *Asia Pacific Disability Rehabilitation Journal* **9**, 4–8.

Pfeiffer, D. (2000). The devils are in the details: the ICIDH2 and the disability movement. *Disability and Society* **15**, 1079–82.

Shakespeare, T. and Erickson, M. (2000). Different strokes: beyond biological essentialism and social constructionism. In *Coming to Life*, ed. M. Rose and S. Rose. New York: Little Brown.

Shakespeare, T. and Watson, N. (2002). The social model of disability: an outdated ideology? *Research in Social Science and Disability* **2**.

UPIAS (1976). *Fundamental Principles of Disability*. London: Union of Physically Impaired Against Segregation.

World Health Organization (1980). *International Classification of Impairments, Disabilities and Handicaps*. Albany, NY: WHO.

4

Concepts of community

Overview

> What life have you if you have not life together? There is no life that is not community.
> (T. S. Eliot, choruses from *The Rock*)

An understanding of the concept of community will be useful for two reasons. First, by clarifying what the term means in isolation, it will provide a framework from which we can begin to understand what rehabilitation in the community involves. This will present an opportunity to define community rehabilitation as it stands in practice today, and highlight the factors that are integral to the notion of community.

The second reason for exploring the term is that with a better grasp of its comprehensive make-up we may be guided in the development of more effective approaches to delivering rehabilitation in this context. With better insight, strategies for delivery can be constructed from the inside out, and it may serve to restore and even recreate community links encouraging greater community integration and participation.

At the core of the concept is the notion of some form of boundary that distinguishes one community from the next. While it is a necessity, ironically it can also prevent full integration with society at large. This is discussed along with a possible solution by way of a successful working model. The chapter ends with an application of the findings to the practical reality of current community rehabilitation. Some tentative recommendations are also made in the light of this overview.

Historical conceptions

In sociological terms, the concept of community and its existence have been assumed for as long as people have been living on the planet. For as long as there are people, there will also be communities. The rise of industrial capitalism was said to have led to the demise of the community. Urbanization was thought to destroy the wholeness of human nature (Gadacz, 1994), leading some to believe that communities were only present in rural settings (Tonnies, 1955). Discussion pertaining to communities is extensive both in health and social sciences literature, but there is general consensus that through being so dynamic and fluid in nature, the concept of community has undergone a significant transformation over the years. How it has changed is encapsulated in the following remark: '... the community is obviously no longer a self-contained, self-sufficient, homogeneous village, but neither has it become an impotent group of unrelated, alienated, anonymous residents with little or no local ties' (Lyon, 1987: cited in Gadacz, 1994).

So while there is still some element of discrete togetherness, it has undergone a change. Change is also apparent within society as a whole, where society is regarded as the body that encompasses all the individual communities. The sheer increase in number of identifiable communities through an acute focus on differences, and deviation from the norm, has contributed to a rather disjointed outlook of society at large. 'Institutionalisation, segregation and the categorisation of people by ability, social class, ethnic origin, or race, gender and age have all contributed to the weakening of social integration and community cohesion' (Gadacz, 1994). Perhaps it is the growing emphasis on differences, as opposed to similarities, that has created this perception of a deterioration of the community.

In summary, while there tends to be agreement towards a noticeable disfigurement in the meaning of community over time, it is in the details of its conceptualization that there are ingredients for dispute. This is reflected in no less than 94 different definitions (Hillery, 1955).

Defining community

Finding a single, universally accepted definition of community has yet to be accomplished. Whether it is possible is unknown; whether it is useful is debatable. Peat (1997) identified three components that engender the concept, based on a definition of community proposed by Helander. They refer to locality, social organization and commonality.

The first component is that of locality. Geographic location is a common thread among many conceptualizations, whereby the community is defined according to geographical boundaries. It does not refer only to the sense of physical space but what is contained within it. Peat described this as a geographical area that contains social structures that meet the physical, psychological and social needs of the majority of its members (Peat, 1997). This construct is a very tangible one, and perhaps the reason why it features so extensively in the literature. It is also the way in which the government facilitates the coordination and delivery of services across the country, using physical boundaries to allocate responsibility to specific authorities.

The second component is that of social organization, whereby a community is made up of a group of people 'linked by history, policies, politics, language or specific needs and implies the involvement of more than just one person' (Peat, 1997). This relates to sharing a lifestyle led according to specific rules or disciplines, and forms the basis for what is known as community 'spirit'.

The third distinction is of a community being created by common interests and characteristics; a sharing of needs, values or culture. This is a dynamic construct, whereby communities are formed via fluctuating interests, that are likely to change over time. Common ties have usually come about through personal choice, and not through fixed characteristics imposed at birth, such as nationality.

Community in context

Rather than searching for the ultimate definition, perhaps greater understanding can be gleaned from a review of its use (Lynd and Lynd, 1929: cited in Jewkes and Murcott, 1996). This will be done through exploring the terms community care, community integration, community-based rehabilitation and community rehabilitation. In so doing it also presents an ideal opportunity to outline the parameters of community rehabilitation in the context of this book.

Community care

Historically, 'community care' was a term coined to reflect the mass movement towards deinstitutionalization of people who were originally segregated because of their differences, be they mental or physical. Today, it consists of a combination of services that enable these people to be supported in their own homes or in smaller residential accommodation. These services are domiciliary in nature, such as home-help, meals on wheels and provision of bathing equipment. The majority of these services are generally classified within the realm of social services, which is why community care should be distinguished from primary healthcare. Even to those people working within the healthcare system this distinction may not be obvious. However, what is agreed is that community care is comprised of support provided outside of institutions and thus the use of the term is geographical in nature.

Community integration

Community integration is a term gaining in popularity. McColl et al. (1998), in a study to investigate the term in relation to the brain-injured population, identified three of the most common conceptions of community integration according to the literature. They are as follows:
1. Relationships with others.
2. Independence in one's living situation.
3. Activities to fill one's time.
Through a qualitative study of their own, McColl et al. (1998) identified nine factors that together were able to define community integration from the perspective of clients themselves. These factors were: orientation; acceptance; conformity; close and diffuse relationships; living situation; independence; productivity; and leisure. The application of community in this context emphasizes the social interactions implicit within the community to the exclusion of any physical restrictions or characteristics.

Community-based rehabilitation

Originally programmes were developed in the South where resources are limited and access to rehabilitation is restricted to urban-based institutions. These programmes were designed to encourage participation by the community members themselves and create a sustainable model of rehabilitation for the future. Community-based rehabilitation programmes are owned and run by the community members themselves to varying degrees. This largely depends on whether they are community initiated or 'grassroots' (where the programme has been developed *by* the community themselves) or community orientated (when it has been developed *in* the community by people outside).

These projects seem to tap into the raw essence of community, especially when they are developed from the grassroots. The community is at the heart of the project, and thus through the project we may learn about the community itself. The uniqueness of each project reflects the diversity of the different communities involved. Where the community is partially defined by physical space, in that members will come from the surrounding area, the boundaries are rarely fixed. Rather the community in this sense is defined by a collective need for services by certain individuals in addition to the network of individuals that provide the support. Thus community in this respect is a picture of togetherness, solidarity and interdependence (see Chapter 8).

Community rehabilitation

The community in the context of CBR conjures images of a cohesive unit, working together towards a unified goal. While it is certainly influenced by geographical location, it is its members who largely define it. In community rehabilitation, greater emphasis is placed on the former, more physical constituents. This is reflected in the following points that attempt to summarize what is meant by community rehabilitation. They refer to:
1. Where it is not.
2. Physical boundaries.
3. Individual perspectives of community.
The primary understanding of community rehabilitation is of rehabilitation that is not delivered in hospitals or institutions. The 'community' in community rehabilitation has been constructed by envisioning where it is not (Jewkes and Murcott, 1996), in the same way that the notion of community care was developed. Despite appearing somewhat vague in its make-up, this conceptualization actually provides an exceptionally accurate basis on which to introduce what is meant by community rehabilitation. It is dependent on physical boundaries inasmuch as they define the areas of exclusion.

Locality is the focus of another aspect that defines community rehabilitation, and indeed, in respect of planned resources a community is usually
defined geographically (Hennessy and Swain, 1997). This point, while it is
also geographically orientated, uses boundaries to isolate areas in which rehabilitation will take place. Whereas it does not explicitly exclude particular
institutions, by defining its boundaries it is inherently exclusive, resulting in
an isolated pocket of activity primarily for political purposes.

Politics is the reason why community rehabilitation is largely regarded
in a geographical way. However, the delivery of rehabilitation depends on
having a population to serve, and geographic features are likely to be of
less significance to individuals themselves. It is more likely that personal
connections constitute a greater impact, as the following statement indicates:
'... lifestyles were largely influenced by social class or stages in the family cycle,
rather than by locality' (Gans, 1967: cited in Compton and Ashwin, 1992).

Individual perspectives are the final, and perhaps the most underestimated,
factor that is relevant to the definition of community rehabilitation. Each
individual has their own personal view of what constitutes their own community (in terms of family, friends, neighbours, social systems, community
activities, organizations, religious belief, etc.) and this directly impacts on
how the individual is reintegrated back into their community. Consequently
the type of social relations within a community determines the choice of the
community interventions that may be used (Borkensha and Hodge, 1969).

Hence, the term community rehabilitation encompasses several facets that
are centralized around geographical markers. Placing equal emphasis on less
geographically defined features of the community, and developing a more
unified understanding of the community within a rehabilitative context, will
expand possibilities for advancing methods of community rehabilitation.

The wider community

Minority groups come together to voice collective needs. They come together
to be heard so that their needs may be met. This is the grounding for a
definition of community, based on similarity of need and an assumption of
homogeneity. Through such mechanisms a minority group, such as disabled
people, can be readily isolated which creates barriers between this group and
society at large. Specialist services are developed for this group, exacerbating
segregation further, making the dividing line ever more defined between

providers of services and the consumers (Gadacz, 1994). The rehabilitative care system becomes dependent on the existence of this isolated group and the relationship between them becomes rigid, stagnant and unhealthy.

The formation of communities in this way can actually be detrimental to the values and principles of such a minority group. Disabled people are demanding equal rights and responsibilities, and yet in expressing their needs have isolated themselves. In realizing that the boundaries that define them can also become barriers to the wider community, the issue of segregation can be addressed. Full participation and inclusion in community life may then become a reality.

Independent living

One way in which to fully understand the concept of community is to learn from a successful working example. A group of disabled students in the University of Berkeley came together in the 1960s and created what is known today as the Independent Living Movement (see Chapter 5). The centres that have arisen as a result represent healthy, integrated and supported communities for disabled individuals because they bring people and organizations together that would otherwise work in isolation. It reflects a community-building activity whereby their values have been incorporated into the structural foundation.

Perhaps it is through such centres that rehabilitation services can penetrate the disabled community in a way that is acceptable to them, resulting in both clinical and cost-effective care. In her analysis of these schemes, Gadacz concluded that returning the person to the community and re-establishing personhood depends ultimately and necessarily for its success on a balanced and integrated working partnership between informal or natural support systems and specialized support systems and specialized formal systems (Gadacz, 1994). Implementing and adapting such a model would potentially provide a means of entering the community without a hypothetical blindfold.

Conclusion

'A central feature of any discussion of meanings of community is seen to be the question of who constructs it as well as when and in what situation' (Jewkes and Murcott, 1996). Community will always mean something different to each individual, thus finding a specific definition is perhaps both impossible and meaningless. Although there are many recurring themes, there are as many disagreements. What one person regards as a community another would not (Jewkes and Murcott, 1996). The concept of community is a very personal and individualized assembly of thoughts and experiences. This suggests that communities are inherently heterogeneous, and not the homogeneous entities that they at first appear to be.

An individual identifies with a particular community so as to address a particular need or set of circumstances (Peat, 1997). What is often overlooked in the conceptualization is that each individual is themselves part of one or a number of self-identified communities. The discrepancy between members' and nonmembers' concept of a community (Jewkes and Murcott, 1996) generates an arena of constant change, dependent on who is doing the constructing and on what grounds. On this basis it would seem that individuality, rather than homogeneity, lies at the core of community, and this may have major implications for the delivery of rehabilitation.

Hospital-based care can be too ritualized, and insensitive to individual need. This may be one reason why opportunities for a transition to deliver services in the community are being examined. They provide a unique opportunity to structure services that not only respond directly to need, but are delivered in the context of an individual's own perceptions of his/her community. To be fully and effectively operational, however, will demand careful planning and negotiation.

'Within the community is an enormous resource of knowledge and goodwill which can be used to help the person who is brain-injured, and the family' (Freeman, 1997). This is not only applicable to those people with brain injury but also to any person within the community. In health and rehabilitation, the community houses a massive wealth of opportunity. The challenge lies in discovering what these opportunities are and how to make them accessible.

In addressing the concept of community this chapter has contributed to an understanding of what is meant by the term community rehabilitation. Specifically it relates to geographical placement, and can be described as rehabilitation that occurs outside of institutions and usually within politically enforced boundaries. Regard for the more qualitative aspects of community, such as personally created constructs of the term (which include social relations and organizations) take second place. This bias towards geographical interpretations of the term should be reviewed. It is common knowledge that the quality and quantity of rehabilitation services differ according to locality. Thus effectiveness of rehabilitation is determined through geographical factors. We need to readdress this balance through a thorough understanding of how social support networks contribute to positive clinical and cost outcomes. Maybe then geographical features will not take priority.

While three aspects have been individually identified to facilitate the understanding of community rehabilitation (where it is not, geographical boundaries, individual perspectives), it is important not to disassociate them in reality. There is a need for a comprehensive understanding and appreciation of the nature of each individual's community, including its diversity, the organizations, boundaries, ties, interactions and social and political frameworks (Peat, 1997). The 'understanding and knowledge of the community is important, not least because of the absence, or existence or potentiality of support networks/systems that are within it' (Hennessy and Swain, 1997).

Before a health professional can effectively enter into the community, a more integrated conceptualization of the community is required. This may be achieved by a quantitative and qualitative examination of all its uses. Of importance, in rehabilitative terms, is to be adaptive and accommodating in the face of diversity, and ultimately have respect for individuality.

REFERENCES

Borkensha, D. and Hodge, P. (1969). Community development: An interpretation. In *Social and Economic Change*. San Francisco, California: Chandler Publishing Company.

Compton, A. and Ashwin, M. (1992). *Community Care for Health Professionals*. Oxford: Butterworth Heinemann.

Freeman, E.A. (1997). Community based rehabilitation of the person with a severe brain injury. *Brain Injury* **11**, 143–53.

Gadacz, R.R. (1994). *Re-Thinking Dis-Ability: New Structures, New Relationships*. Edmonton: The University of Alberta Press.

Hennessy, D. and Swain, G. (1997). Developing community health care. In *Community Health Care Development*, ed. D. Hennessy. Basingstoke: Macmillan.

Hillery, G.A. Jr (1955). Definitions of community: areas of agreement. *Rural Sociology* **20**, 111–23.

Jewkes, R. and Murcott, A. (1996). Meanings of community. *Social Science Medicine* **43**, 555–63.

McColl, M.A., Carlson, P., Johnston, J. et al. (1998). The definition of community integration: perspectives of people with brain injuries. *Brain Injury* **12**, 15–30.

Peat, M. (1997). *Community Based Rehabilitation.* London: WB Saunders.

Tonnies, F. (1955). *Community and Association.* London: Routledge and Kegan Paul.

5

The views of disabled people

Overview

The content of this chapter contains the essence of what rehabilitation should, logically and ideally, be about. Rehabilitation is a service that has been developed for disabled people; thus common sense should dictate that disabled people themselves should be asked what they want out of the service. Unfortunately, due to political and historical influences, this has often not been the case.

Disabled people have been voicing their needs for some time now, but this has largely fallen on deaf ears. Developments within the last few decades have demonstrated that these are not only needs, but they also constitute basic human rights. This in turn has led to some international changes in the legislative framework. Despite growing acknowledgement of their discrimination, many disabled people still feel that the healthcare service fails them. Often needs are assumed, without disabled people being asked directly, which has resulted in ineffective systems of care. This has meant that disabled people have had to find their own solutions to problems. One such solution has been through the development of independent living centres. This service evolved from the principles of the social model of disability (see Chapter 3), and often negates any input by qualified health and social care professionals. The relationship between such centres and traditional rehabilitative institutions varies enormously, often being nonexistent. By combining the academic background of health professionals with the first-hand experience of disabled people themselves, there is enormous scope for establishing a mutually beneficial arrangement. Developing partnerships, by increasing awareness and respect for each other's philosophies, may lead to a better quality of life for disabled people and better use of limited resources. This chapter will discuss these points at length, as well as reviewing the experiences of disabled people directly. First, however, need itself will be defined, along with a discussion about the issues surrounding its assessment.

Definition of need

One way in which 'need' has been defined, and of particular relevance here due to its health-related context, is that formulated by Bradshaw (1977). Bradshaw recognized four different types of need: (1) *felt need* – as perceived by the individual; (2) *normative need* – as defined by an expert; (3) *expressed need* – demand reflected by way of waiting lists and current activity etc.; and (4) *comparative need* – whereby individuals in similar circumstances are presumed to share the same needs. Traditionally, rehabilitation has been driven according to *normative* need, and this is unsurprising considering its medical origins. *Expressed* and *comparative* need have been employed intermittently, being especially useful in quantitative analysis, but they remain predictive in nature, making them rather indirect in their approach. In rehabilitation, assessing *felt* need has been the least well researched of all four types. However it is gaining in status, being widely regarded as the way forward in the rehabilitative arena. However, ways in which to accurately identify this type of need vary enormously, leaving many to question its authenticity. Indeed the result may just be tokenistic to users i.e. *felt* need as interpreted by the professionals.

Assessment of need

Condeluci et al. (1992) examined an interesting study that compared clinical outcome ratings and the values assigned to them by three different parties: the 'survivors'; the family; and 'the payers' (Ferris, 1992). They asked participants to rank the importance of 15 potential outcomes that individuals with brain injury might achieve through rehabilitation on a scale from 1 to 15. They found that the greatest discrepancy between the rankings was between the survivor and the other two groups. 'For payers and professionals, the emphasis for both outcome and value appears to rest with functional, tangible gains. The skills required for walking, talking, and physically doing tasks hold a premium. On the other hand, for families and survivors intangible features such as happiness, autonomy, and equality are of primary importance . . . [survivors] want to be seen as people, and not only as the isolated tasks they are capable of performing' (Condeluci et al., 1992). The differences noted were proposed to be due to variations in motives, such as reducing financial obligations for payers and caregiver burden for families. Consequently, need varies according to who is doing the needing, and it is vital to clarify this in its assessment.

In recent years, there have been increasing numbers of studies to investigate need, largely in the form of need-based assessments. There is a shortage of reliable and effective ways in which to identify need. Focus groups, service statistics, interviews, surveys and questionnaires are all methods by which to identify need. The method chosen will depend on the availability of both financial and personnel resources. However, each method is likely to highlight different aspects of 'need', and caution must be applied in its interpretation. It is difficult to be sure that needs identified through assessment procedures reflect actual need. For example, there is a danger that people will express satisfaction in the absence of informed knowledge about all the options available, or that need based on current activity will not reveal genuine demand. A study that investigated the validity of a questionnaire based upon the Service Quality Model, revealed that its use may be able to make major contributions to rehabilitation care, highlighting patient needs in relation to identified symptoms (Pot, 1999). Alternatively it may be just another illustration of the large discrepancy between the assessment of needs and the underlying need itself; a discrepancy that is brought about because those assessing needs have different agendas from those being assessed.

Some would argue that we do not need to do any more studies of need and that we should start addressing need. This may be true, as long as we know that it is consumer needs that have been identified, and that they have been accurately assessed. However, due to obvious fiscal restrictions, only those needs that are most pressing and highest in priority are likely to be addressed. The problem lies with identifying who should have the right to construct the list of priorities, and hence whose needs are really being met. Power and control still lies very heavily with professionals and funding bodies, resulting in an inadequate representation of consumer needs. The purpose of the following chapter will be to focus on need from a disabled perspective.

Needs or rights?

'... We [disabled people] have been dealt with as a problem in need of special treatment and not as equal citizens with a right to full participation in the social mainstream' (Davis, 1996). Unfortunately many disabled people are deprived of some of their fundamental needs. Considerable activity within the disabled people's movement in recent decades has fought to redress this imbalance. What was once considered to be unmet need is now considered to be a violation of basic human rights. Like feminism and racism before it, disabled people are striving for equality.

'We [disabled people] have pointed out that we need legislation which enables us to take control of our lives, live independently and make a contribution to society. We have warned that until this kind of legislation has been enacted countless millions more pounds will be wasted just keeping us in a state of dependency and second-class citizenship' (Davis, 1996). In voicing their needs, the discrimination that disabled people have faced over the years has become increasingly recognized. This has led to an obligation by governmental agencies to respond by way of enforcing new policies to address this inequality, and to promote disabled people as being active partners in change (Harrison, 1999). The equal rights agenda sits very comfortably with the notion of client empowerment; a key aspect of a professional ethos, which has moved beyond the rhetoric and into practice (Scullion, 2000). However, the rhetoric may be all there about 'people with disabilities' and 'empowering', but in reality there is little evidence that attitudes and practices will significantly change unless they are tied into practical policies (Leach, 1996).

If disabled people are enabled to assess and articulate what they need to achieve a good quality of life, and if the assessment process becomes an effective channel of communication about need – unadulterated by professional assumptions about what need is and how it should be met – then community care policies are much more likely to promote human and civil rights. (Morris, 1993)

Assumption of need

Disabled people 'were socially visible only as patients, clients or welfare/charity cases – under control of medical and other disability-related professionals' (Leach, 1996). It is far too easy to make assumptions about what disabled people want and need, the classic example being the introduction of various charitable foundations. Charitable agencies may appear to be one way of meeting these needs but generally they only serve to accentuate disabled people as victims, thus enforcing their powerlessness and unequal status. Charities have grown to encompass every identifiable medical condition and are in a position of significant power and control (MacFarlane, 1996).

Countless millions of pounds have been and are spent on research into why we are the way we are, on attempts to cure us, or rehabilitate us ... or make us fit into a society designed to serve and perpetuate able-bodied interests. However, when (despite all this effort) we don't quite fit, or can't quite function, or we can't find jobs, millions more pounds are spent on social security, or welfare services, or heart-warming charitable endeavours designed to compensate us in some way for the personal tragedy that has befallen us. (Davis, 1996)

Furthermore 'assumptions that disability necessarily means dependence, nonproductivity, and powerlessness have to be rooted out' (Roberts, 1989). The consequences of such assumptions not only lead to discriminatory attitudes, but also to inadequate systems of provision and extensive inefficiency of resources. The introduction of community care can be used as one such example.

Community care

The principles that should underpin community care, as identified by users and carers themselves, are respect; autonomy; being treated as an individual; recognizing the totality of individual needs; choice; recognition of the work and needs of carers; and partnership. In reality 'community care' still contributes to the view of disabled people as dependent and different, thus reinforcing their social exclusion and marginalization (Priestley, 1999). Even the term 'care' itself implies that disabled people are in need of help, which does nothing to eradicate their unequal status.

The community care initiative was enforced as a response to consumer needs and rights for greater independence and an end to isolation and institutionalization. What has resulted, however, is institutionalization in a different environment (Morris, 1993). Community care, rather than being a response to the needs of disabled people, has really just proved to be an initiative that provides assistance for those working and living with disabled people (Beardshaw, 1988). This has not only accentuated professional domination, but has also exploited the use of informal carers. While the implementation of community care has enabled disabled people to live in their own homes, their reliance on informal carers has actually impeded any further autonomy and limited choices.

'I think the community care philosophy doesn't understand what independent living is . . . They seem to think that community care is about someone being cosy and comfortable, being kept clean. To me that's a step back into the situation of residential care – living in the contained environment of your own home. If you don't broaden it out it isn't independent living' (a user's view: in Morris, 1993). The term 'independent living', in the context of community care policies, has been used to refer to various initiatives that forgo the need for institutions and professional supervision. Independent living, through the eyes of a disability activist, means an entirely different thing altogether, and this forms the basis of the next section.

Independent living

Despite government efforts to identify and address specific demand, there is still a large amount of unmet need. Needs are complex and unique and they are difficult to address within the context of current services for a multitude of reasons. Professional dominance has led to powerlessness on the part of the disabled person. When authority is such that it does not listen to the views of the disabled person then the reality of unmet need is almost inevitable. Financial constraints also serve to prevent needs being fully met. Not only is this due to insufficient funds, but contractual arrangements determine what and how services are delivered, leaving little leeway for responding to consumer needs.

In response to this backdrop of unmet need disabled people have had to find their own solutions. One such solution has been in the form of independent living centres, developed as part of the independent living movement. Independent living centres are places run by, and for, disabled people, based on the philosophy that disabled people themselves are the most informed about their own needs. The concept of independent living was born in the early 1970s by a group of disabled students at the University of California. 'Independent living meant freedom from isolation and institutionalization; it meant the ability to choose where to live, how to live, and how to carry out the activities of daily living that most able-bodied people take for granted' (Roberts, 1989). The principles of the social model lie at the heart of this movement with the primary objective of placing disabled people at the core of planning, implementing and running their own services. User involvement, participation, control and choice are key variables that shape its make-up, resulting in the provision of services on the clients' own terms in direct response to their personal needs, and not that of external funding bodies.

Independent living centres vary worldwide. This variance is noted in the observation that while they are termed 'independent' in the USA, they are called 'integrated' living centres in the UK. The reason for this is found in their respective healthcare policies. The existence of the welfare state in the UK demands that these centres work in association with other statutory agencies, whereas they function more or less independently of the state in the USA. Typical activities of these centres are peer counselling, advocacy and self-help, in addition to lobbying for an accessible environment, for integrated education and the right to employment. The unique issues of the community and the culture in which it is embedded mould the exact activities of each centre.

Financial aspects of independent living

The issue of personal assistance has traditionally been the key focus in the independent living movement because of the great stigma attached to not being able to do things for oneself (Morris, 1993). The introduction of Direct Payments, which enables disabled people to pick and buy their own services is a significant improvement. There is increasing evidence that giving disabled people the cash to pay for personal assistance not only creates a better quality of life but is also a more cost-effective way of meeting personal assistance needs than services provided by the statutory organizations (Morris, 1993).

The option of living at home and receiving a care package with control over who is employed to assist in meeting everyday needs is a relatively new phenomenon. As one disabled person put it: '... disabled people cannot rely on friends and volunteers for the help they need – we must be able to pay for it and be in control of our day-to-day lives and independent of those around us' (Vasey, 1996). However, as revolutionary and beneficial this system has proved to be, in the words of one user: 'It inches you nearer towards a mainstream life but does not allow you to reach it' (Vasey, 1996).

The impact of the Independent Living Movement

'The IL movement is more than a grassroots effort on the part of the disabled to acquire new rights and entitlements; it is also reshaping the thinking of disability professionals and researchers, has spawned new service-delivery models, and has encouraged new research directions' (DeJong, 1979). It has provided alternatives to traditional medical and rehabilitation services, not only advocating individual empowerment, but community change as well. A crucial difference between the independent living philosophy and the rehabilitation model is that services are not limited to short-term need. They are provided for the lifetime of disabled individuals (Roberts, 1989).

Through both qualitative and quantitative research methods, Hutchison and colleagues investigated the impact of independent living centres on the community in Canada. Independent living centres were seen as 'the most reliable and effective source of support for many people with disabilities in the community' (Hutchison et al., 2000). However, they were found to have a bigger impact at the individual level than on the community as a whole. One participant noted that 'they're not reaching the medical community or the government and they don't network with other consumer groups' (Hutchison et al., 1997). In spite of this, they 'have been working hard to collaborate with community agencies to create change, by forming partnerships, educating community groups, monitoring the community's sensitivity to disability issues, and helping to develop new services' (Hutchison et al., 1997). It is clear that independent living schemes have opened a lot more doors for disabled people, but there is still a lot more to be done.

Health professionals and independent living

Many independent living programmes have specific practice arrangements regarding the employment of nondisabled professionals. A study by Bowen (1994) found that of 96 programmes investigated in the USA, only 46% reported using occupational therapy services. This is despite the fact that independence is a concept highly valued by occupational therapists and to assist others in living as independently as possible is a primary goal in their work.

In an international overview of resource centres on disability, 47% of the centres employed occupational therapists, 8% employed speech therapists, 7% employed physical therapists, 4% employed nurses, 4% employed social workers and 1% employed psychologists (Hampton, 1993). Even though the percentage of those providing it is the highest of all the health professions, occupational therapy is still not provided at more than half of all centres that were investigated. This is echoed in the observation that given the choice, some disabled people will choose to employ personal assistants who are un-qualified so that they have no preconceptions about their role and they can train them to meet their own personal needs (Morris, 1993).

In following the principles of independent living, there is a limited role for traditional rehabilitation services, as we know them. 'Rehabilitation is seen as part of the problem, not the solution' (DeJong, 1979). Rehabilitation services have been judged as 'a major disservice to disabled people . . . [and] with the removal of the economic and social barriers which confront disabled people, the need for rehabilitation in its present form would be greatly reduced or eliminated altogether' (Barnes, 1991). This constitutes a considerable threat to the rehabilitative professions. In the UK, where the welfare system encour-ages joint planning with the statutory services, there is scope for some form of compromise. The Derbyshire Centre for Integrated Living works in part-nership with other organizations, aiming to highlight disabling practices and working to enlighten health and social services personnel about the priorities of disabled people (French and Swain, 2001). If rehabilitation professionals and disabled people can join forces, there is a greater likelihood of building effective services that meet the needs of both alliances. This may be explored further through a recruitment practice that encourages applications from disabled health professionals. With these points in mind, it is now time to identify the needs of disabled people, listen to what users of current services are saying and value this experience in its own right.

The value of consumer experience

Professional dominance in the provision of rehabilitation contributes to the doubt about whether disabled people have the ability and knowledge to identify their own needs. A lack of knowledge about their impairment and the services on offer has brought professionals to the conclusion that their clients are unable to accurately express and identify what they need. This may be true within the rigid framework of current service provision, but it ignores another equally important perspective: that of individual experience. Growing amounts of literature are pointing towards the same conclusion; rehabilitation professionals must listen to their clients. 'Rehabilitation professionals need more information about consumers' perspectives on effective and ineffective components of our interventions' (Sabari et al., 2000). It is not enough just to draw on professional experience. 'The major focus in rehabilitation studies has been on the patient's functional recovery as seen by the health professionals . . . what tends to be missing from the research literature are the patients' own subjective experiences' (Cant, 1997). Indeed 'If we are not satisfying those at the core of rehabilitation, there is something seriously wrong . . . We suggest that the perceptions and feelings of services recipients regarding outcomes and their value are as valid as other measures of outcome more commonly performed . . . It is intriguing and perhaps, symbolic that few reviews from this perspective exist in our current literature base' (Condeluci et al., 1992). The following sections aim to present this disabled perspective.

General need

Seven primary needs have been identified by disabled people in Derbyshire (Silburn, 1988). These interacting needs are for information; access; housing; technical aids; personal assistance; counselling; and transport. The same survey showed that disabled people also wanted more generally based community services rather than specific professional services. Another source, that corroborated this finding, revealed that the priorities for disabled people comprise somewhere to live, appropriate care services, mobility, access and opportunity (Swain, 1993). Furthermore, an investigation of local surveys of user groups identified the following factors to be of importance, in order of priority: accessibility; community services; continuity of contact; emotional support; information; evaluation; and provision of equipment (Radermacher, 2000). It is promising to note that all these findings share many features, suggesting that there is some commonality of need. The question is whether these needs are being addressed. The following reports about disabled people's experiences of rehabilitation may begin to answer this question.

Disabled voices

By reviewing this literature and learning what disabled people want from a service, we can attempt to bridge the gap between what is currently provided and what is actually required. Much of this information is extricated from qualitative studies that allow participants to determine the focus and direction of the research themselves or from their own written reports. Thus the majority of the following section will be made up of quotes relating to individual perspectives which remain relatively untarnished by professional interpretation. It is difficult to know where to begin and where to end in sharing the views of disabled people. It is not for the authors to make judgements about which comments are the most relevant or significant. Therefore in documenting what disabled people have said about services, the purpose is for the reader to get a feel for its essence in addition to its specific content. There is little in the way of any additional explanation, as each comment generally speaks for itself. To facilitate its absorption, however, the material is broken up into subsections.

About rehabilitation in the community

What emerged from the data of a study investigating the role of people who received rehabilitation in the community (Abbott, 1999) was that above all, patients and carers valued rehabilitation highly. However, delays and interruptions in services upset service users, particularly when unexplained, and they felt that their views had not been sought or incorporated into the assessment and treatment plans. 'Survivors value the skills leading to independence but place greater importance upon relationships and their acceptance in the community' (Condeluci et al., 1992).

A qualitative report concerning the reflections on rehabilitation by members of a community-based stroke club found that the 'specific issues of major concern to the stroke survivors and their caregivers included a lack of individualised treatment, a tendency for professionals to disregard issues related to stroke survivors' general quality of life, inadequate home care services, and insensitive health care workers' (Sabari et al., 2000). Frustration surrounded the fact that rehabilitation services were concentrated during the first few weeks after the stroke, a time when many of them were not ready to take full advantage of the therapists' expertise. Early discharge programmes are being more widely implemented, with a focal aim of decreasing the length of inpatient stay. 'How can any survivor adapt and learn everything in that brief period of time, while going through confusing changes in body and mind?' (Newborn, 1998). This was said by someone who experienced a stroke, knowing that discharge into the community meant a reduction or cessation of services.

Along with the inadequate approach to issues of intimacy and sexuality, the participants in Sabari et al.'s study were left to feel ill equipped for their transition back to community living. This point was mirrored by an independent report from an individual who had had a stroke herself, in which she commented that 'the skills taught and learned in the early rehabilitation phase do not necessarily transfer to real life' (Buscherhof, 1998). She went on to add that she was 'appalled by the lack of theory and research in the professional literature pertaining to psychological rehabilitation after stroke . . . In today's managed health care environment, the focus of rehabilitation is on cost containment and measurable results' (Buscherhof, 1998).

McKevitt and Wolfe (2000) reported on findings from a study which asked interviewees to identify the main problems they faced and to give their views on what a stroke-specific community service should offer. Participants wanted more information, particularly about the implications of having had a stroke, with ongoing access to therapy. The monitoring of progress was seen to be a gap in current service provision. Participants tended to look to family and friends for support, which conflicted with professional priorities to provide emotional support. The diversity of individual needs, and the range of resources they bring with them, serves to make the identification of a single intervention to solve all problems unlikely. Besides, 'problems identified by participants do not translate directly into needs with ready solutions' (McKevitt and Wolfe, 2000).

'Even if you make it through to life in the community, you are often abandoned. No services, no support. This has been my experience too. Over a long period of time, you learn about the services that are available, but these services are usually fragmented, inadequate and inefficient. People who provide such services often have very little understanding of ABI [acquired brain injury] and the narrow definitions of eligibility mean that you are usually unable to receive any services. In all of the time since my accident, despite threats of institutionalisation, suicide attempts, constant medication and multiple hospitalisations, I've never had any lifestyle support. Never. Not any. And the situation is the same for nearly all the survivors I know' (Sherry, 1999).

About staff

In an investigation of the management of the healthcare needs of 22 severely disabled people living at home, 'there was an ambivalence about relationships developed with health professionals . . . [they] were generally esteemed and respected . . . [however] Dislike and distrust was common if the health professionals showed either by word or by deed that they disagreed with or did not understand the participant's decisions . . . There was a perception that the health professionals often thought the participants were too costly or a bother . . . [and] The lack of knowledge amongst health professionals about the disability was a recurring perception. The health professionals who did receive accolades were the ones who had made personal contact with the participants, had listened to them, had appeared to help them, and had treated them like a friend or equal' (Stephens, 1998).

Likewise, another person noted that 'the importance of a sympathetic and caring staff cannot be overstated. This applies especially to the ancillary staff who, not normally valued for their therapeutic skills, play an undoubtedly important part in this process. They should receive official acknowledgement for this because they are so important in creating the 'normality' that is so necessary for one's mental health . . . [and] I was truly impressed by the calm tireless efficiency of most of my nurses . . . Despite these favourable impressions, a few nurses did strike me as patronising even when they clearly were trying not to be so' (Cant, 1997). Of professional expertise, he concluded: 'I am not convinced anyone really understood what was happening in my brain in a physiological sense, any more than I did' (Cant, 1997).

Therapists 'appeared as a group to be congenitally pessimistic . . . I could understand their reasons for constantly warning you not to expect a complete recovery . . . However, I felt that it would be easier to cope with possible disappointment . . . rather than with the pessimistic deflating contemporary ethos that seemed to permeate the work of physiotherapy and occupational therapy' (Cant, 1997). 'Individual therapists are often disappointed, frustrated and embarrassed by the failures of services as a whole . . . and this embarrassment may explain why delays and interruptions to services are unexplained. It also seems likely that staff are unwilling to encourage service users to express wishes, however appropriate, which cannot be fulfilled because of resource constraints' (Abbott, 1999).

About intervention

'When she was in hospital, she was shown how to do things at home which she wouldn't do at home, because other members of the family would do it, and had always done it. Therefore it was a waste of time . . . the occupational therapist has made the mistake of actually assessing what she thinks you need, rather than what you think you need' (Abbott, 1999). Similarly, for people on medication, 'although the medication was continued, some participants did not think it was beneficial. The medication had often been prescribed some years ago and there appeared to be no monitoring of its continued suitability' (Stephens, 1998).

There was 'no opportunity to ask for alternative solutions [to unfeasible recommendations and] . . . The home care visits, which should have provided such an opportunity, were too rushed and impersonal to meet this need' (Sabari et al., 2000). 'The major preference was for regular physiotherapy . . . but this need was not being met in the way the participants wished . . . the excuses given for not providing this were vague and ambiguous. Several participants felt abandoned by the health professionals, and did not know what to do when a problem arose . . . The other biggest concern was bladder and bowel control . . . All participants would have liked this aspect managed more effectively. The lack of information was another complaint . . . Continuity in the health service personnel was seen as a priority . . . The participants preferred the health professionals to make domiciliary visits, because this meant quality time was given to the individual' (Stephens, 1998).

About psychosocial aspects

'Stroke survivors tended to emphasise how important it was for rehabilitation professionals to pay adequate attention to the social and psychological consequences of stroke after discharge to the community' (Sabari et al., 2000). This point is reflected in a qualitative report on counselling disabled people where 'more often than not it is the client's lack of control over their physical and social environment and not the impairment that causes emotional difficulties' (Oliver, 1995).

About financial arrangements

Funding is a common source of frustration for many disabled people. Not only is there not enough, but it is tied up in contractual agreements with various conditions for use. 'The money spent on my stay there [a home for older adults] could have been put to better use paying for the alterations to my apartment, but I suppose these things come from different budgets' (Janson, 2000). In another story a woman stated that 'she would prefer to be given the money equivalent of their input so that she could purchase all her care from one source. Social services does not seem to have the flexibility to match client and carer satisfactorily, and she is concerned that she has to adjust to different carers from week to week . . . I feel that social services and health will only do what they have to do, and no more' (Swain, 1993). To add to the limitations of the present funding system, 'there was a fear that care could be taken away because financial arrangements could be changed . . . The sheer effort of arranging for treatment or visits of formal health situations was too much for some participants and they sought other ways to solve the problems' (Stephens, 1998).

About perception of impairment

Individual perceptions of impairment range enormously, and this is more than likely going to influence perceptions of rehabilitation and its purpose. 'I was 47 years old when I suffered my stroke . . . it was almost a year since I had become ill' (Janson, 2000). This lady regarded her experience of stroke as of being inflicted with an illness, thus rehabilitation may have been seen as a necessary treatment to get 'well' again. A comment made by another person with stroke emphasized the feeling of loss and the need to establish a new identity: 'I could not accept that I was in disrepair. I had to enter a long grieving process, feeling the 'total' overwhelming loss of the past me' (Newborn, 1998). However, the sense of loss and illness is not always an inevitable consequence of stroke, as a further statement reveals: 'Although I was treated as being seriously ill I did not feel ill in the sense of having the unpleasant symptoms of flu or something similar. I felt perfectly normal within myself . . . but losing my independence and becoming the raw material for many people's jobs was a shock to my sense of normality' (Cant, 1997).

A final remark

'Mr L believed that, in the hope of long-term benefit, he needed in the short term to be responsive to staff's wishes rather than to his own' (Abbott, 1999). This comment illustrates the powerlessness of disabled people within the present system. While in this case, Mr L was willing to take what he could get; many others are taking a different stance. Some will find alternative arrangements, hoping that eventually their grievances will be heard. Although 'disabled people cannot be treated as a homogeneous group' (Oliver, 1995) due to there being a large diversity of opinion, Wendell (1996) has argued that collectively they can still be distinguished from those of nondisabled people.

Towards a partnership

Integrating models of rehabilitation

The rehabilitation goals of disabled people cannot be met by medical rehabilitation services alone, and it is only by integrating them within a network of other services that these goals can be achieved (Fuhrer et al., 1990). The relationship between independent living centres (ILCs) and medical rehabilitation programmes (MRPs) was investigated and the three most frequently endorsed barriers to stronger relationships were conflicting approaches or styles of service delivery, funding of services and conflicting programme philosophies. However, Fuhrer et al. (1990) concluded that 'it appears that ILCs and MRPs are indeed complementary in meeting the multiplicity of needs of persons with physical disabilities.'

This study identified several further initiatives that were attempting to demonstrate effective collaboration between ILCs and rehabilitation services to assure a continuity of services from acute care hospitalization through to community living (e.g. between the University of Michigan model spinal cord injury system and the Centre for Independent Living Serving Washtenaw County). Personal correspondence by the author with an ILC manager in Canada revealed a positive relationship between their centre and nearby medical institutions. The manager was careful to acknowledge that they represented two distinct operations, both with important roles, but it is the way in which they respect, communicate and work with one another that is of importance. Rather than independent living being regarded as a component of community rehabilitation, or conversely, community rehabilitation as a component of independent living, structures are required to amalgamate the two so as no longer to be components of one another but one and the same.

Collaboration between various alliances has also been investigated at the planning level. Sullivan et al. (1997) addressed the issue of consumer involvement through equal representation on Community Health Boards and majority representation on Regional Health Boards in Nova Scotia, Canada. This was based on the notion that individuals within communities would be better able than centralized organizations to assess the health and rehabilitation needs of their constituent members, and would likely hold greater investment in ensuring that health and rehabilitation programmes are implemented and maintained. It was concluded that the success of the system will depend on forming strategies to overcome barriers to full consumer involvement.

Perspectives from the South

Due to pressures from the consumer movement and ongoing cost awareness issues, current methods in community rehabilitation are slowly changing. One modification is the accommodation of elements of consumer participation, adopting an approach more in accordance with models of independent living and community-based rehabilitation. Community-based rehabilitation originated in the South (see Chapter 8) as a result of limited access to professional rehabilitation services. Its primary aim was to provide basic rehabilitative assistance to large numbers of people in the most cost-effective way, relying on partnerships between funding bodies, consumers and the whole community for its success. The emphasis on consumer and community participation is a feature it shares with independent living programmes, which can create the false assumption that they are identical in their aims and ideologies. They are however inherently different. Community-based rehabilitation has no history of associations with any consumer movements, and developed purely as a response to need within a medical context and gross financial restrictions. Power still lies heavily within the hands of the professionals. 'This essential difference has engendered a tension between the two in regard to which is the more appropriate successor to the traditional rehabilitation model' (Lysack and Kaufert, 1994), introducing a competitive edge rather than one of compromise and integration.

The future

'Tesco or Sainsbury's have to provide their shoppers with food they want to buy or go broke. They cannot blame their failure to do this on the poor communication and collaboration between shop assistants, managers, food processors, farmers, transporters and the like, and still hope to remain in business. Yet human service workers do this all the time and do still remain in business' (Oliver, 1991). Supermarket chains and consumers have developed a more symbiotic and equal relationship. Consumers have the choice as to where they want to shop which means that supermarkets must be attuned to the needs of their customers.

Similarly, it is hoped that in developing methods of rehabilitation for the future, rehabilitation practice will incorporate the values of everybody involved, so it too can hope to promote healthy, symbiotic relationships with its consumers. Currently, rehabilitation practice is so entwined in cost control and efficacy, that it can overlook more pressing factors, such as the needs and experiences of its clients. For example, 'although HCH [hospital care at home] is generally perceived as offering increased choice to patients, there is real danger that a preoccupation with cost control might reduce patient choice in the location of treatment' (Marks, 1991). Thus, despite evidence that rehabilitation in the home is cheaper and as effective as hospital care, it does not necessarily imply that it is what people want.

Traditionally, relationships between health professionals and their disabled clients have been unequal, whereby 'professional workers have defined, planned and delivered the services, while disabled people have been passive recipients with little if any opportunity to exercise control...To be truly effective, health and welfare professionals must relinquish their power and control and work closely with disabled people under their direction' (French, 1994). It is not possible to hope that simply by asking people what they think about services will necessarily constitute user involvement. Disabled people need to be at the core of planning and providing their own services, and ways in which to facilitate this process require further exploration.

The growing success of independent living schemes is evidence to suggest that it is an effective model of service provision. However, by gaining in status they threaten to lose sight of their origins, becoming ensnared in the same bureaucratic traps as statutory organizations and entering into the very power relations that they aimed to initially abolish. Only a small percentage of disabled people belong to consumer-directed groups and thus have the authority to make decisions, which endangers an underlying principle of the movement that promotes choices for all. The challenge lies in recognizing the continual tendency toward power inequalities and to attempt an immediate redress (Lysack and Kaufert, 1994).

Further development of rehabilitation services without acknowledging other models, such as independent living, will serve to create a deeper rift between systems of service provision. This is a waste of precious resources. There is no doubt that disabled people want and require rehabilitation services, but by finding ways to integrate the principles of all models, and establishing a partnership, may maximize the benefits. 'Rehabilitation professionals must continuously seek creative and feasible solutions to the problems identified by our clients' (Sabari et al., 2000). The key point is that for disabled people's needs to be met, they must first be listened to and understood.

REFERENCES

Abbott, S. (1999). Planning and implementation of care: the patient's role. *British Journal of Therapy and Rehabilitation* **6**, 398–401.

Barnes, C. (1991). *Disabled People in Britain and Discrimination: a Case for Anti-discrimination Legislation.* London: Hurst.

Beardshaw, V. (1988). *Last on the List: Community Services for People with Physical Disabilities.* London: King's Fund Institute.

Bowen, R.E. (1994). The use of occupational therapists in independent living programs. *American Journal of Occupational Therapy* **48**, 105–12.

Bradshaw, J. (1977). The concept of social need. In *Planning for Social Welfare Issues, Models and Tasks*, ed. N. Gilbert and H. Specht. Englewood Cliffs, NJ: Prentice Hall.

Buscherhof, J.R. (1998). From abled to disabled: a life transition. *Topics in Stroke Rehabilitation* **5**, 19–29.

Cant, R. (1997). Rehabilitation following stroke: a participant perspective. *Disability Rehabilitation* **19**, 297–304.

Condeluci, A., Ferris, L.L. and Bogdan, A. (1992). Outcome and value: the survivor perspective. *Journal of Head Trauma Rehabilitation* **7**, 37–45.

Davis, K. (1996). Disability and legislation. In *Beyond Disability: Towards an Enabling Society*, ed. G. Hales, pp. 124–33. Bristol, PA: The Open University.

DeJong, G. (1979). Independent living: from social movement to analytic paradigm. *Archives of Physical Medicine and Rehabilitation* **60**, 435–46.

Ferris, L. (1992). *The Outcome Rating Scale: a Survivor Perspective.* Pittsburgh, PA: United Cerebral Palsy.

French, S. (1994). Disabled people and professional practice. In *On Equal Terms*, ed. S. French, pp. 103–18. Oxford: Butterworth-Heinemann.

French, S. and Swain, J. (2001). The relationship between disabled people and health and welfare professionals. In *Handbook of Disability Studies*, ed. G.L. Albrecht, K.D. Seelman and M. Bury. Thousand Oaks, CA: Sage Publications.

Fuhrer, M.J., Rossi, D. and Gerken, L. (1990). Relationships between independent living centers and medical rehabilitation programs. *Archives of Physical Medicine and Rehabilitation* **71**, 519–22.

Hampton, M.M.K. (1993). An international overview of resource centres on disability. *American Journal of Occupational Therapy* **47**, 725–30.

Harrison, J. (1999). Health care access and equality for disabled people. *British Journal of Therapy and Rehabilitation* **6**, 380–3.

Hutchison, P., Pedlar, A., Lord, J. et al. (1996). The impact of independent living resource centres in Canada on people with disabilities. *Canadian Journal of Rehabilitation* **10**, 99–112.

Hutchison, P., Pedlar, A., Dunn, P. et al. (2000). Canadian Independent Living Centres: impact on the community. *International Journal of Rehabilitation Research* **23**, 61–74.

Janson, L. (2000). Sweat, patience, and perseverance. *Topics in Stroke Rehabilitation* **6**, 60–3.

Leach, B. (1996). Disabled people and the equal opportunities movement. In *Beyond Disability: Towards an Enabling Society*, ed. G. Hales, pp. 88–95. Bristol, PA: The Open University.

Lysack, C. and Kaufert, J. (1994). Comparing the origins and ideologies of the independent living movement and community based rehabilitation. *International Journal of Rehabilitation Research* **17**, 231–40.

MacFarlane, A. (1996). Aspects of intervention: Consultation, care, help and support. In *Beyond Disability: Towards an Enabling Society*, ed. G. Hales, pp. 6–18. Bristol, PA: The Open University.

Marks, L. (1991). *Home and Hospital Care: Redrawing the Boundaries.* London: King's Fund Institute.

McKevitt, C. and Wolfe, C. (2000). Community support after stroke: patient and carer views. *British Journal of Therapy Rehabilitation* **7**, 6–10.

Morris, J. (1993). Community care or independent living. In *Independent Lives?: Community Care and Disabled People.* London: MacMillan Press.

Newborn, B. (1998). Quality of life for long term recovery in stroke. *Topics in Stroke Rehabilitation* **5**, 61–3.

Oliver, J. (1995). Counselling Disabled People: a counsellor's perspective. *Disability Handicap and Society* **10**, 261–78.

Oliver, M. (1991). Multispecialist and Multidisciplinary – a recipe for confusion? 'Too many cooks spoil the broth'. *Disability Handicap and Society* **6**, 65–8.

Pot, J.W.G.A. (1999). Development of a needs assessment system in rehabilitation. *International Journal of Rehabilitation Research* **22**, 155–9.

Priestley, M.A. (1999). *Disability Politics and Community Care.* New York: Jessica Kingsley Publishers.

Radermacher, H. (2000). *Review of the Regional Neurological Rehabilitation Services.* Newcastle-upon-Tyne: Newcastle City Health NHS Trust.

Roberts, E.V. (1989). A history of the Independent Living Movement: a founder's perspective. In *Psychosocial Interventions with Physically Disabled Persons*, ed. B. Heller, L. Flohr and L. Zegans, pp. 231–51. New Brunswick, NJ: Rutgers University Press.

Sabari, J.S., Meisler, J. and Silver, E. (2000). Reflections upon rehabilitation by members of a community based stroke club. *Disability and Rehabilitation* **22**, 330–6.

Scullion, P. (2000). From exclusion to inclusion: a key role for rehabilitation staff. *British Journal of Therapy and Rehabilitation* **7**, 105.

Sherry, M. (1999). Re: Brain Injury. Disability research mailbase. http://www.jiscmail.ac.uk/cgi-bin/wa.exe?A2=ind9910&L=disability-research&P=R22407. 25 Accessed June 2001.

Silburn, R. (1988). *Disabled People: their Needs and Priorities.* Nottingham: Benefits Research Unit, Department of Social Policy and Administration, University of Nottingham.

Stephens, J. (1998). The Needs of Severely Disabled People Living at Home: how do Severely Disabled People Living at Home Manage their Health Care Needs? *Action Aid Disability News* **9**, 51–5.

Sullivan, M.J.L., Irving, C., Jamieson, P., et al. (1997). Involving consumers with disabilities in Nova Scotia's reformed health system. *Canadian Journal of Rehabilitation* **10**, 307–14.

Swain, P. (1993). Helping disabled people – the user's view. *British Medical Journal* **306**, 990–2.

Vasey, S. (1996). The experience of care. In *Beyond Disability: Towards an Enabling Society*, ed. G. Hales, pp. 82–7. Bristol, PA: The Open University.

Wendell, S. (1996). *The Rejected Body: Feminist Philosophical Reflections on Disability.* New York: Routledge.

6

Outcome measures and research in the community

Introduction

Measurement and research are key components in the rehabilitative engine. Their ongoing contribution feeds the knowledge base, which not only informs practice and attempts to improve upon it, but also raises the profile of rehabilitation within the medical spectrum, and ultimately wider society. Where it is used as an assessment of efficacy and evaluation, it can justify a need for a specific intervention and monitor progress over time. Such results can satisfy audit criteria, reassure providers and funders of services, as well as aid resource allocation.

As well as being useful, research is essential towards establishing, developing and maintaining effective rehabilitative services. Research and measurement can be carried out in numerous ways and at many different levels. With the steady transition of rehabilitation services into the community, many traditional forms of research and outcome measure are no longer appropriate. It is for this reason that it is necessary to examine the different forms of research and measurement in rehabilitation today, and how they can be applied to the community setting. Some outcome measures have been specifically designed for application in the community, but widescale use is in its infancy. This chapter aims to discuss some of the issues surrounding measurement and research in the community.

Qualitative and quantitative research

The word *qualitative* implies an emphasis on processes and meanings that are not rigorously examined, or measured (if measured at all), in terms of quantity, amount, intensity, or frequency. Qualitative researchers stress the socially constructed nature of reality, the intimate relationship between the researcher and what is studied, and the situational constraints that shape inquiry... In contrast, quantitative studies emphasise the measurement and analysis of causal relationships between variables, not processes. (Denzin and Lincoln, 1994)

In medical settings research has been designed, directed, administered and statistically analysed by the researcher, often in quantitative and objective ways. This has been the dominant research paradigm of the field. It often makes several assumptions about its sample population; the most obvious being that the factors under scrutiny can be quantified at all. Qualitative research has its roots in the social sciences, tending to focus on subjective data. In a medical context it is considered by many to lack scientific rigour.

Qualitative researchers tend to use historical narratives, first-person accounts, life histories and biographical and autobiographical materials, among others. Quantitative researchers, on the other hand, use mathematical models, statistical tables and graphs, and often write about their research in impersonal, third-person prose (Denzin and Lincoln, 1994). Due to a generally longer, more time-consuming process, qualitative research involves smaller study groups that do not have to be randomized. Hence, while quantitative methods may elucidate types and trends of behaviour, qualitative measurement can be used to explore why people behave in a certain way, and the meaning behind it.

Quantitative research

The essence of quantitative research is the measurement and quantification of observable data. Quantitative methodologies use a systematic and predefined process for gathering and analysing numerical data, which in theory is collected in a value-free environment. Quantitative methodology used to be seen as the gold standard for research but in recent years the value of qualitative techniques has been increasingly emphasized in clinical research. Quantitative techniques are nearly always practised in laboratory settings and are an ideal mode for research into, for example, drugs and surgical techniques. In a community setting there are often a number of confounding variables, which make quantitative research difficult to perform in isolation and there is often value in combining both quantitative and qualitative techniques in community research projects. Quantitative research will normally rely on a hypothesis, which can be tested in an objective fashion. Whereas the essence of qualitative research is the interaction between the researcher and the subject, quantitative research strives to distinguish objectively between the subject and the researcher. Detachment is the essence of quantitative research whereas participation is the essence of qualitative research. The avoidance of research involvement should help guard against biasing the study towards that individual's own perceptions and values.

Types of quantitative research

There are a number of types of quantitative research, including descriptive, correlational, quasi-experimental and experimental work.

Descriptive research

Descriptive research, as the name would suggest, at its simplest involves the description of objective data. Such data can be collected in descriptive studies by a number of means, including questionnaires, interviews and direct observation. Obviously these techniques can be used in qualitative research but tend to be more structured when used in quantitative work. The use of closed (fixed alternative) questions in the questionnaire design, for example, would be used more than open-ended questions. Observation techniques, whilst more common in qualitative research, can also be used quantitatively. Observers would make particular use of check lists and rating scales so that the behaviour of events that are observed can be organized, structured and analysed.

Correlational research

Correlation studies are not universally accepted as a form of quantitative research. However, the basic premise of this type of study is to determine a relationship between variables. The quantifiable data from descriptive studies are frequently analysed in this way. For example, a researcher may look for differences between two groups with regard to satisfaction or usage of a particular service parameter.

Experimental and quasi-experimental research

Experimental research is often the most appropriate for testing a cause-and-effect relationship and is generally accepted to be the most powerful quantitative methodology. Experimental research tests hypotheses. An hypothesis, for example, may be made that a particular treatment A reduces long-term disability more effectively than another treatment B. A randomized set of participants (preferably a large group) are subject to the influence of treatment A (the independent variable) and response is measured (the dependent variable). The other group is subject to intervention B and the results compared. A key to experimental techniques is that individuals should be randomly selected for exposure to each (or sequentially both) variable. If such complete randomization is not possible then a quasi-experimental design may be used. This is often appropriate if it is impossible, either practically or ethically, for individuals to be randomly allocated to either treatment conditions or if it is unacceptable to be given no treatment or a placebo in a control situation. Semlyen et al. (1998) used a quasi-experimental design, for example, in a recent study of the efficacy of multidisciplinary rehabilitation. This was a study designed to measure the efficacy of a multidisciplinary rehabilitation team for those who attended a regional rehabilitation centre. Comparison was made with individuals discharged from a neurosurgical unit, with traumatic brain injury, who were not referred to the rehabilitation centre but were sent to a nonrehabilitation hospital environment or sent straight back home. Complete randomization of referrals was not possible on an ethical or practical basis as referral often depended on bed availability and the overall opinion of suitability by the rehabilitation team. In these circumstances a quasi-experimental design was adopted with robust quantifiable outcome measurement in both groups but with acceptance of the fact that both groups may have been different at the time of transfer. Indeed in this example, the group referred to the rehabilitation centre was somewhat more disabled than the group discharged elsewhere.

Control

Quantitative research depends on reducing the influence of extraneous variables, which are not being studied at the time of that particular experiment. This control over the research variables can be achieved in a number of ways.

Sampling

It is clearly important for the sample of subjects that are to be exposed to the independent variable to be as representative as possible of the population being studied on such matters as age, sex, social class, educational attainment, etc. Ideally the sample population should be completely randomized into a group that receives the experimental variable and a group that does not (the control group). Obviously nonrandom allocation methods, such as individuals volunteering to enter one group or the other, may well bias the outcome and prevent generalization of the results. However, the ideal of random sampling is not always obtainable in research. The population, for example, may be too large and logistics of the research may require that only a subsample is used in the research. Systematic sampling may be necessary. This will involve the subjects being chosen based on the position on a list. For example, every fifth name could be selected in a list of people with multiple sclerosis and then this subsample invited to participate in the study. In smaller groups such systematic sampling may still produce groups with a relative bias. Thus, stratified sampling may be required. The whole population may, for example, be split up into age, sex or level of disability. Random sampling would then take place in each subgroup in order that the eventual experimental population is representative of the population as a whole.

Research design

The eventual aim of quantitative research is to include as large a population as possible so that the quantifiable results can be analysed and the results of such analysis would then be generalizable to the population as a whole. Thus, particular care needs to be given to the nature of the randomization process and the size of the eventual experimental groups.

The actual design of the experiment will clearly vary according to the nature of the intervention and the circumstances of the study. The two (or more) randomly selected groups could simply be exposed in parallel to the treatment variable or the control situation (parallel group design). Alternatively one group could be exposed to the experimental intervention whilst the other group acts as a control for a period of time. The groups could then swap with the original control group then receiving the intervention whilst the original experimental group acts as the control (cross-over design). Sometimes one group can act as its own control receiving an intervention and then a control intervention at a later (and/or earlier) stage. There are obviously other design strategies to suit particular situations. If at all possible the experimental group should not be aware of the type of treatment received – whether it is the experimental condition or the control condition. Ideally the researcher should also not be aware of the experimental condition in order to avoid potential researcher bias. If neither the participant nor the researcher are aware then such studies are called double-blind. If the participants are not aware but the researcher does know the experimental condition then these are termed single-blind studies and if all parties are aware of the experimental condition then these are termed open studies. The double-blind, placebo-controlled study is the most robust form of experimental design.

Measurement

The nature of quantitative research is accurate measurement of the experimental variable. Obviously many outcomes can be measured. At one end of the scale are impairment measurements. It may be possible to test, for example, the range of motion after particular antispastic intervention or a physiotherapy technique. However, in a community setting measurement is often more desirable at the level of activity and even at the level of participation. The more the outcome measure moves towards the participation end of the scale then the more difficult is accurate quantifiable measurement, as so many extraneous variables will often come into play. This is often the challenge of community rehabilitation research and why, in a community setting, quantitative and qualitative research often need to go hand in hand.

A discussion of measurement scales that have been used in community rehabilitation is reserved for the end of this chapter. There are a significant number of scales appropriate to different research circumstances and the reader is referred to the excellent review of the subject by Wade (1992). However, in any research, including community research, the measurement scale used should be appropriate to the research circumstance and fulfil a number of criteria. First it is important to understand the nature of the scale. There are four types of measurement scale: nominal, ordinal, interval and ratio.

Nominal scales do not scale items along any dimensions but rather label them. Variables such as gender or ethnicity are common nominal variables. They are simply data that have a category label and therefore should be subject to descriptive interpretation rather than statistical analysis.

Ordinal scales order people, objects or events along a continuum. However, it is important to emphasize that there is no precise measurable difference between the ranks on an ordinal scale. As an example the Ashworth Scale, commonly used in the measurement of spasticity, is an ordinal scale and the difference between an Ashworth score of one and two is not the same, in any measurable sense, as between a score of three and four (Pandyan et al., 1999).

Interval scales are similar but provide equal differences between the scale points. A common example is the Celsius scale of temperature where a 10-point difference has the same meaning anywhere along the scale. Interval scales can be subject to more rigorous statistical analysis and robust parametric tests can be used.

Finally, ratio scales are the same as interval scales but have a true zero point. Examples of ratio scales are length, volume, time and so on. Ratio scales can also be subject to robust statistical analysis.

It is quite a common mistake in research terms for ordinal scales to be subject to parametric statistical analysis (e.g. mean, standard deviation, etc.), although such analysis is invalid. Nonparametric statistics are the only valid statistics that should be used on ordinal scales. Whatever scale is used, however, it should be both valid and reliable.

Validity

Validity underpins the experimental research process and refers to the degree to which an instrument measures what it is supposed to be measuring. There are a number of different concepts concerned with validity.

External validity concerns the question of whether the findings of the study can be generalized beyond the sample from which they were derived.

Population validity relates to whether the results of a particular study can be applied to different groups of people. This often depends on the sampling, which should have ensured that the population studied was representative of the population as a whole. Ecological validity concerns whether the results of the study could apply in other places and contexts. This concept is often important in community studies. As an example, if a particular physiotherapy technique improves walking in the research laboratory it is important to ensure that such a technique will also improve walking abilities in a real home when a carpet may be used instead of a smooth laboratory floor.

Other concepts focus on internal validity, which is about the nature of the scale itself. There are three important dimensions to internal validity – *content validity*, *criterion validity* and *construct validity*. *Content validity* is concerned about the extent to which the measure adequately covers the various dimensions of the concept under investigation. All aspects of the concept should be covered by the measurement scale and not just one particular aspect. If an intervention, for example, purports to improve independent mobility then all aspects of independent mobility should be measured in the scale, including indoor and outdoor mobility, on different surfaces and stairs, etc. *Criterion validity* can be further split into two different concepts. Concurrent validity means that a particular scale has been put up against an existing and well-accepted measure – the gold standard. Predictive validity assesses the degree to which a measure can predict a future event – such as the risk of future pressure sores or the degree of recovery from traumatic brain injury. Finally, *construct validity* refers to the extent to which a scale is measuring the underlying theoretical constructs. If, for example, the scale purports to measure pain associated with spasticity then it should measure both pain and spasticity as the two are the essential components of the underlying construct.

Reliability

In addition to a scale being valid it should also be reliable. The concept of reliability is concerned with the extent to which a measure produces consistent results. Some degree of inconsistency is present in all measurement techniques but such inconsistency should be kept to a minimum in any experimental procedure. There are two particularly important concepts – inter-rater and intra-rater reliability. The former refers to the fact that two separate observers measuring the same event should produce the same results. In other words there is no ambiguity in the testing procedures, which might be subject to different interpretations between different experimenters. Intra-rater reliability refers to the test/retest stability of the measure. The same observer should get the same results if the test is repeated over time (assuming that the underlying variable is not changing over time). There are various statistical analyses that are possible to measure reliability that are beyond the scope of this chapter.

Finally, it is useful for a scale to be simple and easy to administer as well as being understandable and communicable to others – both other researchers and other interested parties. It is unlikely that a given measure fulfils all the necessary validity and reliability criteria. However, it is important to choose a scale that has at least been through some degree of vigorous review. It is pointless to use a scale that has not been shown to be valid and reliable as this would defeat the object of quantifiable experimental research.

In summary, quantitative research can produce robust and generalizable answers to quantifiable research questions. The problem in community research is that many problems are not readily quantifiable and thus not readily measured. It is probably fair to say that health research has been rather too obsessed with quantitative techniques to the detriment of qualitative techniques. Anyone with an interest in research in a community setting should be familiar with quantitative methodology but should have an equal familiarity with qualitative methods and be prepared to use either methodology at the appropriate time.

Qualitative research

Whereby quantitative research is essentially deductive, qualitative research is inductive (Pope and Mays, 1995). Instead of starting with a hypothesis and testing it, the research theory may emerge as the study evolves (this is known as 'grounded theory' methodology). While the researcher should not impose her/his own knowledge upon the agenda, at the same time she/he is a fundamental link in the research system. The extent to which the researcher is involved varies, and this shapes the nature of the research and the subsequent findings. For example, in observational fieldwork, a researcher may or may not disclose her/his identity. If identity is disclosed then the researcher may act as a form of participant (Mays and Pope, 1995b). In addition to their specified role, it is vital that the researcher has an intimate understanding of the setting, and pays particular attention to the language used and its meaning.

If carried out well, qualitative research has good face validity. It is possible to further safeguard validity by feeding back the findings to participants for comments, or by running focus groups to discuss the findings. By doing so this further generates data production. Practice such as this makes it difficult to distinguish between data analysis and its collection, which is a common feature of qualitative study. Findings from such research are not necessarily representative of the population. Participants are chosen to facilitate an exploration of the focus of the research, and hence key informants are selected. However, attention must be given to minority opinion and views that do not concord with the researcher's overall theory, as well as the general findings (Kitzinger, 1995).

Qualitative research has been criticized (e.g. for lacking generalizability and reproducibility, and being subject to researcher bias) but there are ways in which to ensure a more rigorous process. If another trained researcher can follow the same methodology and come to the same general conclusion then it should be sufficient. Systematic data collection and analysis, adequate documentation, meticulous records, copies of transcripts and appropriate computer software can all facilitate this process. Like all research, method-ological processes must be theoretically justified.

There are several ways in which qualitative data can be collected. Where they each share the same underlying principles, they also have unique charac-teristics that make them particularly suitable for specific occasions. *Observational studies* take place in natural settings and require systematic and detailed observation of behaviour and talk. In this way it helps to over-come the discrepancy between what people say and what they actually do that other more verbal methods can not reach (Mays and Pope, 1995*b*).

Interviews are a very popular qualitative research technique, being espe-cially useful at tapping into individual biographies (Britten, 1995). The ways in which they are conducted fall into three main categories; structured in-terviews often involve a questionnaire framework, whereas semistructured interviews use open-ended questions, and in-depth interviews cover one or two issues in great detail and are usually led by what the interviewee says. In their interaction interviewers need to be particularly sensitive to language and key concepts. They also need to be aware of how they are perceived by the interviewee, and in what way this might impact on the interview. Attaining a healthy locus of control is a great skill, along with minimizing other common pitfalls associated with conducting interviews (e.g. distractions, interpreter bias etc.). Of particular importance is the setting in which the interview takes place: ideally the interviewee should be given the choice, and being at home is often the most comfortable option.

Focus groups are a 'form of group interview that capitalizes on commu-nication between research participants in order to generate data' (Kitzinger, 1995). The group format enables people to explore concepts, generate their own questions and pursue their own priorities. This can also encourage par-ticipation from those people who may not be comfortable in one-to-one situations, and can also facilitate discussion surrounding more taboo areas. However, any individual voices or opposing views may be lost in the body of group norms. Careful consideration regarding group composition, its size, the setting, the presence of a facilitator and having an opportunity to follow-up on an individual basis afterwards is essential. If these factors are addressed then focus groups can be invaluable sources of data, particularly suited to the study of attitudes and experiences.

Consensus techniques are another qualitative research instrument commonly adopted in health services research. Two of the most familiar are the Delphi process and the nominal group technique (Jones and Hunter, 1995). They provide a way of dealing with conflicting scientific evidence, which avoids common problems associated with group decision making. All participants have the opportunity to provide opinions about an issue, to consider the opinions of others, and to rank them in order of personal importance. During every 'round' the participants are able to change earlier decisions, until a consensus has been met at the final stage. This method enables health providers to come to decisions about situations where there may be too much or too little relevant information.

The last method to be described is not exclusively qualitative. *Case studies* use multiple investigative methods, which may be qualitative or quantitative, leading to greater construct validity (Keen and Packwood, 1995). They are best suited to explore complex questions in equally complex circumstances, such as those found in real-life settings. Attention to detail is essential in a case study; not only in its design and the selection of methods, but also in choosing the site. Its interpretation involves value judgements, and hence to maximize confidence in the findings analysis needs to be highly systematic. The use of such studies is likely to increase in the healthcare setting, as the issues involved in rehabilitation begin to address more and more complex and broader issues. If there is no single truth, as qualitative research assumes, then having multiple perspectives on phenomena would seem to be requisite (Bogdan and Biklen, 1982).

Combining quantitative and qualitative research

Historically, the distinction between quantitative and qualitative research has often been overemphasized. There are benefits of both qualitative and quantitative research paradigms, as they ask and answer different questions. Thus it would seem that they should be complementary (Pope and Mays, 1995), working together towards a partnership-based framework that echoes the ethos of rehabilitative practice elsewhere. Traditional quantitative methods, such as randomized controlled trials, are often the most appropriate means of testing the effect of an intervention or treatment, but a qualitative exploration of beliefs and understanding is likely to be needed to find out why the results of research are often not implemented in clinical practice (Jones, 1995). Furthermore, subjective perceptions are often needed to fill in the gaps left by traditional objective assessments (Whiteneck, 1994).

In 1994 a large-scale national survey of hospital patients in the UK was undertaken by Bruster et al., and typically it followed a very quantitative ideology. It was later criticized by Pound and Ebrahim (1995) for lacking any validity, particularly because the patients were not asked about their own views on the outcome of their treatment. In-depth interviewing and content analysis – methods that accord with the qualitative framework – were recommended as a prelude to designing questionnaires in the future (Pope and Mays, 1995). In this way qualitative research could be used to inform the quantitative component of the study. This represents a sequential design; one of four ways in which clinical research can employ a multimethod design.

Miller and Crabtree (1994) describe three other methods of employing qualitative and quantitative methodologies in combination. They are based on concurrent, nested or combination designs. Concurrent designs bring together the results of two independent studies that have been conducted concurrently on the same study population. Nested designs represent a system whereby qualitative and quantitative research can be conducted within the same single study. Like the sequential design, each research strategy can inform the other, but within the nested design there is an ongoing and dynamic exchange of information. In a combination design, some or all of the designs described above can be integrated in various ways.

These methods of combining qualitative and quantitative research have also been called triangulation (Pope and Mays, 1995; Fielding and Schreier, 2001). This refers to an approach to data collection in which evidence is deliberately sought from a wide range of different, independent sources and often collected by different means (Mays and Pope, 1995a). Udo Kelle (cited in Fielding and Schreier, 2001) describes triangulation as more of a metaphor than a precise concept, as its meaning has become lost over time. As a result he has identified three different models of triangulation: the validity model; the complementarity model; and the trigonometry model. It is the latter that emphasizes the necessity to have a combination of methods in order to gain any picture of a phenomenon at all.

Qualitative and quantitative research paradigms do not then have to be incompatible. A greater understanding and respect of the scope of both methodologies, and a willingness to engage in exploring this relationship could lead to more methodologically sound measurement techniques and ultimately more meaningful results. By combining many different research paradigms greater depth and breadth may slowly be attained, but the truth may always elude us.

Outcome

Doing research, whether it be quantitative, qualitative or a combination of both, has many advantages. However, this is only true if it is carried out in appropriate ways. The problem, of course, lies in identifying what is appropriate and what is not. Validity and reliability are two such qualities that have been known to differentiate between effective and ineffective research instruments. Unfortunately, obtaining validity and reliability does not always mean that administering the instrument is worthwhile. It might also be impractical, lacking in scope, irrelevant or inapplicable in a certain context. If it purports to measure outcome, it may make assumptions about what a positive outcome entails. But what is outcome anyway? Who decides what is a positive outcome? Who decides what and how to measure? Who measures it? Who interprets the results?

These questions have infiltrated the research domain and challenged the way in which research has traditionally been carried out, especially in the world of science. As described more fully in Chapter 5, Condeluci et al. (1992) express considerable surprise at the lack of literature from a client's perspective, suggesting that outcome measures incorporating these views are just as valid as any others that are more commonly performed. Condeluci et al. reviewed several studies, one of which compared the views on outcome of three different parties: 'survivors'; their family; and the 'payers' (Ferris,

1992). They found that the biggest discrepancy lay between the perspective of the 'survivors' and that of the other two groups. 'Survivors' tended to value less tangible features, such as happiness, autonomy and equality more highly. This led to the conclusion that the definition of 'outcome' may deserve expansion to include these less tangible constructs. There is a need to be more open and exploratory about what constitutes a 'good' outcome and the ways in which it will change according to time, place, company and setting.

Outcome in community rehabilitation

Traditionally, outcome measures in rehabilitation have been developed to monitor progress, particularly in acute settings. They have focused on individuals at the level of impairment and activity (as defined by the ICIDH; see Chapter 3), providing an objective measure irrespective of the environment. While this can inform the medical profession about how severe an impairment is, it lacks any appreciation of how the individual him/herself perceives and copes with it, especially in a natural environment. Successful rehabilitation outcomes constitute more than, for example, how much an individual can score on a scale that assesses daily living skills. Similarly, even if an individual is found to have the ability to walk, it does not mean that they will.

Most rehabilitation professionals appreciate this discrepancy but are ill equipped to measure factors of greater global significance (Whiteneck, 1994). As rehabilitation moves into the community the limitations of outcome scales become more critical, and traditional research techniques are even less able to target what matters. Complex global concepts such as 'handicap' or 'participation' may be more difficult to measure, but this is no reason not to do so (Whiteneck, 1994). 'Handicap' or 'participation' (as defined by the ICIDH) is influenced not only by the severity of the impairment, but also by societal limitations and individual characteristics. This makes it a key rehabilitation outcome in need of closer examination.

Investigating the factors that facilitate discharge (community re-entry) and community integration need to take account of the priorities and preferences of clients and their families. Furthermore, not only is there a need to know if problems are resolved, but whether communities are responsive to the needs of these people. In the community the focus of intervention shifts to another dimension. Not only is there an emphasis on the long term, but also priorities for individuals extend beyond the parameters of health and move into relatively unexplored territory of education, housing and employment needs. The difficulty associated with measuring such global concepts goes some way to explain why there are so few consistently used instruments in the community.

Outcome measures

In a review of the use of standardized outcome measures in 182 rehabilitation centres in the UK, 140 (77%) of them collected at least one standardized measure (Turner-Stokes and Turner-Stokes, 1997). The most common measures of global disability were the Barthel index, the Functional Independence Measure and/or the Functional Assessment Method (FAM). At least one or more of these were employed by 123 of the centres. The Nottingham Extended Activities of Daily Living (EADL) scale, the London Handicap Scale and the General Health Questionnaire (GHQ) were also routinely used in about a fifth of the centres. A wide variety of instruments were employed across the sites, indicating that there was no obvious measure suitable for all settings and services. What the researchers did conclude was that the most popular measures could be used to provide a framework for the future collection of data in this field.

Even though popularity alone does not prove that particular instruments should be administered, the findings of this review are useful in as much as they highlight both the range and the inconsistency with which outcome measures are used. There is no ultimate measure, and a selection may be of more clinical use. In the light of this the following section takes the opportunity to explore what has materialized in the way of outcome measures specifically designed for a more community-orientated approach. This is not meant to be a comprehensive review of instruments that have been used, but rather a platform from which to explore the potential of community-based assessments further.

Northwick Park Care Needs Assessment

Although the Northwick Park Care Needs Assessment (NPCNA; Turner-Stokes et al., 1999) is not specifically a measure of community outcome, it can be administered in hospital at admission and discharge and used to estimate the care needs of individuals with severe and complex impairments when they return to the community (Nyein et al., 1999). It takes into account the time required for supervision as well as for physical help, and covers care needs across a wide range of dependency. By estimating care needs in terms of total care hours, this can also inform the costs and planning associated with care packages. Interviews provide the necessary information to score up the assessment. In hospital this is done with the nurse responsible for the patient's day to day care, and subsequent interviews in the community are with the disabled person and main carer together.

Community Outcome Scale

The Community Outcome Scale (COS) developed by Stilwell et al. (1998) was originally designed for the practical use of rehabilitation teams themselves, and not for research purposes. Using both qualitative and quantitative techniques, it records and classifies problems by way of semistructured interviews and then estimates the impact that these problems have on different dimensions of independent living. The four dimensions are mobility, engagement, occupation and social integration. After details of the interview have been analysed by a computer program, each individual obtains a score on each dimension. Lower scores are associated with better outcomes. Practitioners can use it as a method for classification, problem resolution and identification of goals. Managers can use it to identify the types of existing problems, knowledge of which can inform planning and care packages and track the success of interventions. Thus, it can be used not only as a research instrument, but also as a method by which practitioners can audit their service and monitor client pathways.

Community Integration Questionnaire

The Community Integration Questionnaire (CIQ; Willer et al., 1994) focuses on three dimensions: domestic integration, social integration and productivity. It can be completed by self-report or with the assistance of a close other, familiar with the individual's health status and social activities. Although it has good psychometric properties, it lacks sensitivity because of its short length (15 items), and it is recommended that it only be used as part of a more comprehensive assessment (Wood and Worthington, 1999). Considering that a single definition of community integration continues to elude both researchers and service providers alike, it would not be surprising to also find shortcomings associated with its assessment. In a qualitative study to elucidate what community integration consisted of from the perspective of people with brain injuries, it found no less than nine factors (McColl et al., 1999). The study proposed the possibility of a hierarchy, whereby issues at the most basic level, such as home and family, needed to be addressed before the more broad issues of occupation and orientation.

Craig Handicap Assessment and Reporting Technique

The Craig Handicap Assessment and Reporting Technique (CHART; Whiteneck et al., 1992) was specifically designed to measure the extent of handicap (as defined by the ICIDH) in individuals within a community setting. It uses measurable and behavioural terms (i.e. uses quantitative data only) to compare such individuals with the norms of able-bodied members of society. Thus the extent to which the roles, activities and relationships do not match the accomplishments of disabled people's peers is taken to reflect the disadvantage (Dijkers et al., 2000). The CHART is administered as an interview or survey, consisting of 27 questions that are based on the same dimensions of handicap as described by the WHO (1980). These are dimensions of occupation, physical independence, mobility, social integration and economic self-sufficiency. Each item is assigned with different weightings according to the value placed on them by the general population. In addition to having sound psychometric properties, this objective assessment of handicap also has the potential to be used as a method of programme evaluation (Whiteneck et al., 1992).

Quality of life measures

The literature on quality of life contains well in excess of 100 definitions and models and is too vast for any one study to fully assimiliate (Cummins, 1997). There is general agreement that quality of life implies a combination of both objective and subjective variables that are based on normative values and values of individual respondents respectively. Cummins emphasizes the necessity to refer to the general population to develop a construct of quality of life because health-based constructs tend to be overly restrictive, medically dominated and focus on the negative aspects of pathology. According to Cummins, quality of life consists of seven different domains: emotional well-being, health, intimacy, material well-being, productivity, safety and place in the community. Cummins reflected these domains in three parallel versions of the Comprehensive Quality of Life Scale (CumQol), which measures both subjective and objective data (e.g. Cummins, 1993). There are a number of other quality of life scales that have been developed over the years and each have their own proponents. It is not possible or desirable in the context of this chapter to discuss the details of various quality of life measures, but it is nevertheless important to emphasize the key role of using an accepted quality of life measure if one is looking at the overall impact of a community rehabilitation scheme on the life of the individual participants. A scale needs to be chosen that reflects the particular parameters required for that audit or research project. Occasionally researchers are more interested in health-related quality of life. Such standard measures as the Short Form Health Survey (SF–36) or the Health Related Quality of Life Scale (HRQol) may be helpful. However, other projects may need to look particularly at other dimensions. For example, it may be important to assess the needs of families in their own right (Tyerman, 1999). This could be done through careful administration of selected structured interviews and family and marital rating scales. What constitutes a desirable outcome will vary enormously from family to family. Other projects may require more detailed evaluation of vocational outcome. This may include a simple assessment of return-to-work rates but should often include some rating of role satisfaction in the work environment. Once again there are a number of scales to choose from and the reader is referred to other texts (Wade, 1992; Cummins, 1997; Turner-Stokes and Turner-Stokes, 1997; Wood and Worthington, 1999).

Other factors influencing research

Rehabilitation research is driven by a number of factors. Improving individual clinical outcome by providing more effective services is high on the agenda. Developing and administering outcome scales is one way to monitor success, but there are other factors that also need to be taken into consideration.

Cost

'Just as lifetime outcomes must be examined, so must lifetime costs' (Whiteneck, 1994). Whether within a NHS framework, or a largely privatized system, there is a market for cost-effective services. In the USA, where the private system creates a very competitive market, financial strategies become integral to the treatment plan (Papastrat, 1992). An accurate portrait of outcome can determine the running costs of rehabilitation, which is vital to the financial sponsor. Considering the competitive nature of service provision, accurate outcome measurement is likely to benefit both their own service (i.e. in attracting more clients if the price is right) and the job of financial assessors (who need to account for all the costs over time).

Legal requirements

As part of health service frameworks, research plays an important role. In the UK, for example, audits are a matter of routine to ensure high-quality services. Legislation documenting equal human rights for all, lies at the heart of such advances, which means that providing effective services is not only desirable but also enforceable by law. If consumer rights, equality and partnership become even more significant, methods to generate more consumer-based research will become a necessity.

Ethics

Before any research can proceed, it needs approval from an ethics committee. Through such a process, it aims to ensure that the participants in a study are not going to be exploited in any way, and that their health will not be endangered. While this procedure is obviously necessary, its success is dependent on the standards by which the committee make their judgements.

Disability research

'Disability' research refers to research that has been carried out according to the principles of the social model of disability. It is not an all-inclusive term to describe all the research that has ever been done in the field of disability. This is an important distinction to make, as the majority of research that has been referred to in this text will not be placed in such a category.

Traditionally, research has been owned and directed by the researcher, and rarely tends to be relevant or directly beneficial to disabled people. This begs the question, in whose interests is this research in? Obviously the majority would like to say it is for disabled people themselves. However, it often remains inaccessible to lay people and acts only as fodder for academic scrutiny.

The fundamental principle underlying disability research is that disabled people are considered to be the experts, and hence research should be controlled and coordinated by disabled people themselves. According to Moore et al. (1998) disabled people are entitled to a number of rights in relation to disability research. The authors suggest a preliminary list would include rights of access to the process of research (planning, carrying out, dissemination), entitlement to set agendas, to describe one's own experiences and to have personal experience valued; rights to confidentiality, ownership of data, to ask for account to be taken of one's views in implementation of policy and practical changes arising from research, the right to understand the nature of the research and to challenge and reject research.

Although much of disability research is qualitative, Barnes (1992) advocates that it can also be quantitative as long as it is approached from an emancipatory perspective. Disability research challenges much of traditional rehabilitative research, representing an alternative, not necessarily mutually exclusive, way of carrying out research with disabled people. It would be in the best interests of rehabilitation researchers to at least be aware of the principles that underlie disability research, for this would broaden its scope and impact considerably.

Research in partnership

Some disabled people would deny that there is a place for nondisabled researchers in disability research (Branfield, 1998). Branfield states that any attempts at justification for this are doomed to fail. In his response, Duckett (1998) stated that by discriminating and excluding would-be supporters, the disability movement itself fails to see people as equals and consequently reinforces the notion of oppressive practice. It would seem that there is a need for some form of common ground or neutral territory on which disabled people, professionals and researchers can proceed.

Clearly research is an important part in the rehabilitative agenda but if participants and/or disabled people are being 'violated' then it is the responsibility of the discipline to fully investigate these allegations. No one can claim to know more about disability than disabled people themselves. Likewise, one could argue that no one knows more about research than researchers. If the skills and resources of researchers were to be 'at the disposal of disabled people' (Barnes, 1992) this could form the basis of a new partnership.

Conclusion

As rehabilitation moves into the community so too does the context in which research is carried out. Traditionally, research instruments and techniques in rehabilitation have been designed to monitor quantitative variables in controlled environments in very objective ways. This is no longer sufficient to fully appreciate and understand the wealth of dynamic constituents that comprise the notion of rehabilitation in the community.

Instruments that measure single factors in isolation that are judged in relation to a specific norm have limited value. Likewise, attempts to assess more complex factors without some form of systematic procedure are unlikely to be able to appreciate the full spectrum of interacting variables. Both approaches have viable theoretical foundations, but alone they lack substance. To begin to assess more global concepts, such as community integration and quality of life, the adoption of a combined approach, gaining multiple perspectives of the same phenomena, may prove to be a more effective tool for exploring rehabilitation in the community.

REFERENCES

Barnes, C. (1992). Qualitative research: valuable or irrelevant. *Disability Handicap and Society* **7**, 115–24.

Bogdan, R. and Biklen, S. (1982). *Qualitative Research for Education: an Introduction to Theory and Methods*. Boston, MA: Allyn and Bacon.

Branfield, F. (1998). What are you doing here? 'Non-disabled' people and the disability movement: a response to Robert F. Drake. *Disability and Society* **13**, 143–4.

Britten, N. (1995). Qualitative interviews in medical research. *British Medical Journal* **311**, 251–3.

Bruster, S., Jarman, B., Bosanquet, N. et al. (1994). National survey of hospital patients. *British Medical Journal* **309**, 1542–6.

Condeluci, A., Ferris, L.L. and Bogdan, A. (1992). Outcome and value: the survivor perspective. *Journal of Head Trauma Rehabilitation* **7**, 37–45.

Cummins, R.A. (1993). *The Comprehensive Quality of Life Scale – Adult*, 4th edn (ComQol – A4). Melbourne: School of Psychology, Deakin University.

Cummins, R.A. (1997). Assessing quality of life. In *Quality of Life for People with Disabilities*, 2nd edn, ed. R. Brown, pp. 116–50. Cheltenham: Stanley Thornes.

Denzin, N.K. and Lincoln, Y.S. (1994). Introduction: entering the field of qualitative research. In *Handbook of Qualitative Research*, ed. N. Denzin and Y. Lincoln, pp. 1–17. Thousand Oaks, CA: Sage.

Dijkers, M.P.J.M., Whiteneck, G.G. and El-Jaroudi, R. (2000). Measures of social outcomes in disability research. *Archives of Physical Medicine and Rehabilitation* **81** (Suppl. 2), S63–80.

Duckett, P.S. (1998). What are you doing here? 'Non disabled' people and the disability movement: a response to Fran Branfield. *Disability and Society* **13**, 625–8.

Ferris, L. (1992). *The Outcome Rating Scale: a Survivor Perspective*. Pittsburgh, PA: United Cerebral Palsy.

Fielding, N. and Schreier, M. (2001). Introduction: on the compatibility between qualitative and quantitative research methods. *Forum: Qualitative Social Research* **2** (1).

Jones, J. and Hunter, D. (1995). Consensus methods for medical and health services research. *British Medical Journal* **311**, 376–80.

Jones, R. (1995). Why do qualitative research? *British Medical Journal* **311**, 2.

Keen, J. and Packwood, T. (1995). Case study evaluation. *British Medical Journal* **311**, 444–6.

Kitzinger, J. (1995). Introducing focus groups. *British Medical Journal* **311**, 299–302.

Mays, N. and Pope, C. (1995*a*). Rigour and qualitative research. *British Medical Journal* **311**, 109–12.

Mays, N. and Pope, C. (1995*b*). Observational methods in health care settings. *British Medical Journal* **311**, 182–4.

McColl, M.A., Davies, D. and Carlson, P. (1999). Transitions to independent living after ABI. *Brain Injury* **13**, 311–30.

Miller, W.L. and Crabtree, B.F. (1994). Clinical research. In *Handbook of Qualitative Research*, ed. N. Denzin and Y. Lincoln, pp. 340–52. Thousand Oaks, CA: Sage.

Moore, M., Beazley, S. and Maelzer, J. (1998). *Researching Disability Issues*. Buckingham: Open University Press.

Nyein, K., Turner-Stokes, L. and Robinson, I. (1999). The Northwick Park Care Needs Assessment (NPCNA): a measure of community care needs: sensitivity to change during rehabilitation. *Clinical Rehabilitation* **13**, 482–91.

Pandyan, A.D., Johnson, G.R., Price, C.I.M. et al. (1999). A review of the properties and limitations of the Ashworth and modified Ashworth Scales. *Clinical Rehabilitation* **13**, 373–83.

Papastrat, L.A. (1992). Outcome and value following brain injury: A financial provider's perspective. *Journal of Head Trauma Rehabilitation* **7**, 11–23.

Pope, C. and Mays, N. (1995). Reaching the parts other methods cannot reach: an introduction to qualitative methods in health and health services research. *British Medical Journal* **311**, 42–5.

Pound, P. and Ebrahim, S. (1995). National survey of hospital patients. *British Medical Journal* 310, 938–9.

Semlyen, J.K., Summers, S.J. and Barnes, M.P. (1998). Traumatic brain injury: efficacy of multidisciplinary rehabilitation. *Archives of Physical Medicine and Rehabililitation* 79, 678–83.

Stilwell, P., Stilwell, J., Hawley, C. and Davies, C. (1998). Measuring outcome in community-based rehabilitation services for people who have suffered traumatic brain injury: the Community Outcome Scale. *Clinical Rehabilitation* 12, 521–31.

Turner-Stokes, L. and Turner-Stokes, T. (1997). The use of standardised outcome measures in rehabilitation centres in the UK. *Clinical Rehabilitation* 11, 306–13.

Turner-Stokes, L., Nyein, K. and Halliwell, D. (1999). The Northwick Park Care Needs Assessment (NPCNA): a directly costable outcome measure in rehabilitation. *Clinical Rehabilitation* 13, 253–67.

Tyerman, A. (1999). Outcome measurement in a community head injury service. *Neuropsychological Rehabilitation* 9, 481–91.

Wade, D.T. (1992). *Measurement in Neurological Rehabilitation.* Oxford: Oxford University Press.

Whiteneck, G.G. (1994). Measuring what matters: key rehabilitation outcomes. *Archives of Physical Medicine and Rehabilitation* 75, 1073–6.

Whiteneck, G.G., Charlifue, S.W., Gerhart, K.A. et al. (1992). Quantifying handicap: a new measure of long-term rehabilitation outcomes. *Archives of Physical Medicine and Rehabilitation* 73, 519–26.

Willer, B., Ottenbacher, K.J. and Coad, M.L. (1994). The Community Integration Questionnaire: a comparative examination. *American Journal of Physical Medicine and Rehabilitation* 73, 103–11.

World Health Organization (1980). *International Classification of Impairments, Disabilities and Handicaps: a Manual of Classification Relating to the Consequences of Disease.* Geneva: WHO.

Wood, R.L. and Worthington, A.D. (1999). Outcome in community rehabilitation: measuring the social impact of disability. *Neuropsychological Rehabilitation* 9, 505–16.

7

Evidence base for community neurological rehabilitation

Research in rehabilitation

The growing realization is that rehabilitation does not have to be delivered in institutions. Thus the potential for rehabilitation in the community is being proposed and implemented as a viable alternative to traditional methods of rehabilitation. The potential advantages include greater convenience for clients, a familiar environment, involvement of family members and the costs curtailed by not having to provide accommodation. However, this option may be more time-consuming, expensive in terms of therapy time, difficult to coordinate and too much family involvement may be counterproductive (Rice-Oxley and Turner-Stokes, 1999). By delving into the possible opportunities and charting what investigations have already been made, the balance between these advantages and disadvantages may be found.

This chapter aims to consolidate all the research relating to community rehabilitation, and provide a definitive resource to aid further development. It aims to highlight the gaps in the research, and will address accusations that there is a lack of research to confirm the efficacy of rehabilitation in the community (Lafferty, 1996).

Inclusion criteria

Although the studies included in this evaluation will refer to people with a range of neurological impairments, it is apparent that the majority of the literature focuses on stroke rehabilitation. At times it will be pertinent to refer to studies that are not exclusively neurologically based because the findings and models used may aid discussion and understanding. Care has been taken to include studies that employ sound methodological techniques, however, occasionally studies will be included for alternative merits.

Process of evaluation

The evaluation of the present literature surrounding community rehabilitation will be addressed within a number of different sections. This does not represent real differences between the studies themselves but serves to make their assessment more meaningful and manageable. Thus they will be differentiated according to the seemingly different models of rehabilitation they employ. The first is by way of community teams, which appear to be the most common method by which rehabilitation is delivered in the community. Sections will follow on care management, individual therapeutic input, nursing intervention and specialist outreach. Three further studies will be described separately as they fail to fall into any of the above categories. Methodological processes are fodder for criticism and this will be a subject for discussion, following the evidence presented in each section. The chapter then ends by summarizing the literature findings, and presenting some recommendations for the future of community rehabilitation research.

The evaluation – multidisciplinary teams

There appear to be three main stages at which community teams enter into the rehabilitation process as highlighted by the available literature. The first is often referred to as 'hospital at home' and it aims to provide rehabilitation in the home as a direct alternative to hospital admission, negating the need for any inpatient care. The second concerns people who are already receiving hospital treatment, and focuses on reducing the time of admission. This is referred to as 'early discharge' (as well as sometimes being known as 'hospital at home'). The third point at which community teams provide a service is when people are already established in their homes, do not need any acute medical intervention but may benefit from further rehabilitation input. The boundaries between these three stages are by no means fixed but they serve to facilitate the following literature evaluation.

Hospital at home

Hospital at home schemes that act as an alternative to hospital admission will be discussed first. They are defined as 'a service that provides active treatment by health care professionals, in the patient's home, of a condition that otherwise would require acute hospital inpatient care, always for a limited period' (Shepperd and Iliffe, 2000). Of interest is the differentiation between schemes that are community based and those that are hospital based, whereby the former build on existing community resources, the latter provide an outreach service with hospital staff making domiciliary visits.

Forty-nine out of 96 general practitioners (GPs) in a district in the south-west of England were given the opportunity to refer their acute stroke patients to a nurse-led multidisciplinary home care service or, if they preferred, to hospital in the normal fashion (Wade et al., 1985). The acute stroke patients of the remaining 47 GPs formed the control group, and they had access to standard hospital and community services. It must be emphasized that the study did not dictate the location of care, and the GPs made all the clinical decisions. An interdisciplinary team, which consisted of a district nurse, a physiotherapist, an occupational therapist, a speech therapist and a social worker, provided rehabilitation at home to the trial group. Although the team was based in the hospital it only provided rehabilitation in the home. A large number of people were recruited (over 400 in each group) and at the end of 6 months the authors found no difference in functional recovery and emotional adjustment between the two groups, nor any differences in the stress levels of carers. Even though the trial group had significantly more participants at home, it had a slightly higher hospital admission rate for stroke and used 10 902 bed days as compared with 10 511 for the control group. This result raised doubt about expanding domiciliary services to reduce hospital use.

Although this trial, one of the earliest of its kind, erred on the cautionary side of delivering rehabilitation in the community, the apprehension surrounding its success may have been to its detriment. There may have been reluctance by participating health professionals to refer or discharge individuals home until recovery was complete. Another limiting factor of the home-care service design may have been its similarity to the services already available to the control group. Nowadays methods of community rehabilitation, being less alien phenomena, are better developed and more likely to reach their full potential.

For those people with inevitable acute care needs in the future that live in the community, the provision of a hospital at home scheme represents 'a proper target for the evaluation of home-care delivery systems as alternatives to the traditional health-care approach' (Pozzilli et al., 1999). To investigate this, Pozzilli and colleagues compared hospital at home care with routine hospital care for people with MS. The home-care multidisciplinary team included three neurologists, a urologist, a psychologist, a specialist in rehabilitation medicine, a physiotherapist, a nurse, a social worker and a coordinator. Access to the team was via a telephone operator who would in turn contact the appropriate specialist to arrange a home visit. At 1-year follow-up, although there was an increase in client satisfaction with hospital at home care, there were no significant differences in health outcome between the two groups. As well as being a 'popular alternative' to hospital care, it was found that only a few clients required out-of-hours assistance, which would lead to substantial savings. However it would be unwise to conclude that this would reduce costs in the long run because hospital at home schemes open avenues to people who would otherwise not be receiving healthcare services.

An observational study carried out on patients with acute conditions to investigate the feasibility of avoiding hospital admission altogether suggested that hospital at home should be regarded as an 'additional rather than alternative source of care' (Wilson et al., 1997). They concluded that due to the team structure in this particular study it meant that this procedure created an extra work load for GPs and was perhaps not viable, despite being as clinically effective. In the trial that followed the findings were more promising (Wilson et al., 1999). Of 199 people referred to hospital at home by their GP (largely for cardiovascular and respiratory diagnoses), 102 were randomized to the scheme and the rest were allocated to hospital inpatient care. The scheme ran for a maximum of 14 days for each person, providing 4–24 hours of care a day by a team of nurses, a physiotherapist, an occupational therapist, generic healthcare workers, and a cultural link worker. While the scheme was nurse led, the GP maintained medical responsibility. At a 3-month follow-up assessment it was found that there were no clinically or statistically significant differences in outcome. Hospital at home resulted in significantly shorter lengths of stay and this did not lead to a higher rate of subsequent admissions. While this was a positive result, further trials were recommended to investigate the contribution of hospital at home in the management of specific conditions. Iliffe (1998), too, noted that while paediatric hospital at home schemes are well established, caution is advised before substituting hospital at home for all diagnostic groups.

Early discharge

Early discharge schemes (the second identified stage at which community teams intervene) may offer some form of compromise for people who require acute care. They do not negate the need for hospital care, but aim to reduce the admission time. Generally studies have shown that early discharge teams do reduce admission times and can provide a cost-effective alternative to hospital care (Rodgers et al., 1997; Rudd et al., 1997; Coast et al., 1998; Richards et al., 1998; Wilson et al., 1999). However, in one study, for people with orthopaedic conditions, although costs were reduced per day compared with those of standard inpatient care, the length of time enrolled in the programme was longer and thus it was not economically effective (Hensher et al., 1996). This fuels the necessity to evaluate schemes according to diagnosis and cost.

Obviously, cost is not the only deciding factor. While it is important to keep the costs down, clinical outcome and client satisfaction are the critical variables. In a London study, 136 people with stroke were discharged after an average stay of 12 days and received rehabilitation at home for 3 months whilst 126 people remained in hospital for about 18 days and thereafter continued outpatient hospital-based treatment. The total therapy time received by each group was equal, but the intervention group received it at home from a team coordinated by a consultant physician. At 12 months there were no differences between the two groups with regard to activities of daily living. The only difference found was that people in the intervention group were more satisfied with the hospital care that they did receive. The authors concluded that early discharge was as clinically effective as conventional hospital care, in addition to reducing costs in terms of the use of hospital beds and being acceptable to patients (Rudd et al., 1997; Beech et al., 1999).

In Newcastle upon Tyne 92 individuals who were medically stable at 72 hours poststroke were randomized into two groups; one receiving early supported discharge and the other conventional care (Rodgers et al., 1997). The median length of stay in hospital was 13 days for the early discharge group with a median stay of 22 days for the control group. The community-based team was involved with individuals for a median of 9 weeks. The control group continued to receive hospital then standard outpatient rehabilitation. At 3 months after stroke no differences were found between the two groups in terms of functional ability, handicap, health status, carer stress, readmission rate and mortality. However, the early-discharge group did participate more in activities of daily living than the control group. A cost analysis illustrated that the cost of the discharge team was balanced by reduced cost following the shorter length of hospital stay (McNamee et al., 1998).

Similar conclusions were reached in Stockholm. This was a similarly designed study whereby the early-discharge group received 3–4 months of continued rehabilitation at home (Widen Holmqvist et al., 1998). At 6-months follow-up there were no statistically significant differences in patient outcome (von Koch et al., 2000). However, a more detailed analysis suggested a positive effect of home rehabilitation on social activity, activities of daily living, motor capacity, manual dexterity and walking. Death or dependency in activities of daily living was 24% in the intervention group compared with 44% in the control group. There was a reduction in hospital days from an average of 29 days in the control group to just 14 days in the home rehabilitation group. Further investigation into the use of healthcare, the impact on family caregivers and patient satisfaction revealed that 'early supported discharge with continuity of rehabilitation at home, using goal-directed functional activities based on the patient's personal interests, should be the rehabilitation service of choice of moderately disabled stroke patients' (Widen Holmqvist et al., 2000). However this study, along with that of Rodgers and colleagues (1997), lacked an adequate sample size (n = 81) and thus longer and larger multicentre trials are required to assess the generalizability of the results and long-term cost-effectiveness.

In instances when sufficient numbers of participants were able to satisfy statistical scrutiny the outcome was still the same (Richards et al., 1998). A total of 241 elderly, hospitalized people who were medically stable were randomized to receive hospital at home care or routine hospital care. The service at home provided healthcare by a nurse-coordinated team, discharge from which occurred when community services could take over ongoing management. Despite the length of stay in hospital for those receiving routine care being shorter (by 62%) than the time of contact for those in the hospital at home scheme, effectiveness and acceptability was similar for the two groups at 3 months. Hospital at home, even though it was longer in duration, proved to be less costly (Coast et al., 1998) and it was also found to increase the participants' perceived involvement in decision-making.

In summary, early discharge from hospital with specialist rehabilitation at home does seem to be feasible without an increase in readmission rates or increased stress to carers (specifically for those people with stroke). Such early discharge seems to be as effective as conventional care. These teams produce significant reductions in bed usage. This will save costs, which can potentially be used to offset the costs of the community rehabilitation team itself. For those people with other diagnoses, the outcome is less clear.

In the community

The final stage in which teams impact on the rehabilitation process is for those people who do not or no longer require any acute medical treatment but still would benefit from therapeutic support. Such rehabilitation can be given within a hospital setting, in various day-centre settings or within the client's own home. It is in this section that evidence regarding the efficacy of team rehabilitation delivered in the home will be examined. This can either be in the form of community-based teams, or via teams based in institutions that travel into the community. The latter are often referred to as 'outreach' programmes. Sometimes the distance travelled to the community from urban centres is substantial, necessitating the organization of a mobile clinic, and this will be discussed separately in the 'specialist outreach' section.

Programmes in the community tend to be much more client-directed and specifically tailored to the needs of individuals themselves and their families. Adults who had sustained a traumatic brain injury between 3 months and 20 years previously, were randomly allocated to a group receiving either intervention by a multidisciplinary outreach team or written information about other local resources (Powell et al., 2002). The treatment group received an average of two therapy sessions a week for 27 ($+/-$ 19) weeks and this was shown to benefit clients by increasing their independence in self-care, improving their organizational aspects of daily living and aspects of psychological well-being, as well as decreasing 'disability'. These effects extended beyond the period of direct treatment. No differences were noted between the groups in time spent in productive employment or socializing.

Short-term intervention (12 weeks) by a community stroke rehabilitation team resulted in significant improvements in adults under the age of 65 with regard to patient-reported performances, satisfaction and activities of daily living (Plant et al., 2000). The team, managed by a coordinator (physiotherapist), consisted of physiotherapists, occupational therapists, speech and language therapists and a rehabilitation assistant, all of whom were working on a part-time basis. The right to choose the location of therapy (outpatient or home) was valued highly, with many preferring to have physiotherapy within an outpatient setting. Despite the small numbers involved (n = 18), this study highlights that rehabilitation may be more effectively delivered in a combination of settings, dependent on what therapy is being provided.

In another study of stroke rehabilitation, 43 people who remained at home following their stroke were either referred for rehabilitation at home by a consultant-led team, or were provided with the usual outpatient services that a client might expect to receive (Wolfe et al., 2000). The community team comprised therapists from speech, occupational and physiotherapy, making a maximum of one daily visit each, within the 3-month trial period. Community therapy support for patients not admitted to hospital was shown to be 'feasible', based on the results obtained at 1 year. Unfortunately the sample size was not sufficient to confirm statistical significance, concluding that at least 300 participants would have been required to obtain more conclusive results in terms of clinical or cost effectiveness. This has been the case in many studies of its kind (e.g. Rodgers et al., 1997; Widen Holmqvist et al., 1998) and although they are 'useful pilot studies ... [they] do not provide conclusive evidence for clinicians and healthcare planners on how to provide care' (Wolfe et al., 1998).

The impact of longer-term care is not well documented in the literature, and current services fall short of providing support beyond the period of initial rehabilitation (Jones et al., 2000). By not placing a time limit on intervention, an American study that investigated a community-based neurorehabilitation programme for people with brain injuries was able to further inform our understanding of the efficacy of rehabilitation teams (Pace et al., 1999). A core treatment team consisted of a medical director (physician), nurse case manager, programme director and clinical director. Further therapy was provided by a mobile treatment team of occupational and physical therapists, speech pathologists, behavioural psychologists, special educators and rehabilitation technicians. This home-based rehabilitation programme focused on 'real-world' outcomes relating to wherever the individual lived, worked and played, and a committed family member was an obligatory part of the scheme. Individualized outcome planning resulted in great variations in the intensity, length and cost of programmes (the length varied from 2 to > 21 weeks, and the intensity from 1 to 551 hours). Findings showed that 77% of individualized outcome goals were achieved at discharge, and these were 'generally maintained' at 6 and 12 months following treatment. While the number of weeks in the programme did not predict total therapy hours there was a general decline in hours from admission to discharge. This study demonstrated that a home rehabilitation team facilitated the achievement of individualized goals, in addition to adequately satisfying both family and funder. However, without a randomized-controlled design, and no standardized home-based assessment in existence, it makes it difficult to put these findings into perspective and compare them with other research efforts.

These are not the only studies that have incorporated a team structure into the delivery of rehabilitation in the community. Bernabei et al. (1998) found that elderly people who received multidisciplinary rehabilitation in the community organized by a care manager were less likely to be admitted to hospital and if they were, it was appropriately delayed. Goldberg et al. (1997) found that elderly individuals benefited from having rehabilitation via a treatment team after 6 months, but it was not retained at 12 months. Both these studies will be discussed at greater length in the care-management section, and attributing this outcome to the presence of a rehabilitation team (as opposed to the care manager) must be done with caution.

Discussion

The studies that have been carried out have shown that community team rehabilitation is as effective as rehabilitation delivered in other more traditional settings, and thus is a feasible alternative. There are indications of its superiority in specific areas, such as increasing an individual's activities of daily living, but without further investigation and more methodologically sound studies these cannot be confirmed. Thus it 'might be wise to wait just a little longer before giving hospital at home the green light' (Iliffe, 1998).

In addition to the paucity of literature there are many other factors that contribute to the difficulty in evaluating and comparing the effectiveness of this particular model of rehabilitation. They include differences between studies in terms of methodological design, study aims, team structure and the team ethos itself. Methodological design is the subject for much criticism in the field of literature reviews and it is common to any study. Therefore this will be incorporated into the final discussion at the end of the chapter. Of more interest here is to look closely at the variables in team structure and activity that might impact on rehabilitation outcome. For example, there is a distinct difference in 'team' working between clients who just have *access* to therapists, from those who are at the heart of interdisciplinary working. By investigating these variables it may direct our attention to the key factors that determine team effectiveness and thus better rehabilitative outcomes.

Rehabilitation teams varied widely across the studies reviewed. They varied in terms of membership, base, ethos, extent of 'joint' working and family involvement, and leadership (if at all). In some studies teams had an initial team visit/meeting from which intervention was planned and delivered by a selection of other appointed therapists (Hakuno et al., 1996; Pace et al., 1999). Some teams appeared to have regular weekly meetings (Rodgers et al., 1997; Rudd et al., 1997; Pace et al., 1999; Wolfe et al., 2000) with a lot of close contact and joint working, while other teams appeared not to assemble at all. In one study a client had contact with individual team members via a telephone operator (Pozzilli et al., 1999), making the client the only point of contact for team members. Some teams appointed care managers and key workers. This either negated the need for team members to meet or was viewed as an additional characteristic of team working. The care manager was usually a nurse or physician, and they usually took the role of team leader. However, clinical responsibility for each client was usually that of the GP, especially if they were involved in the study (Wilson et al., 1997; Bernabei et al., 1998; Richards et al., 1998).

Team membership consisted of a range of representatives from many disciplines. Some were made up of physio-, occupational and speech therapists alone, whereas others involved physicians, nurses, rehabilitation assistants, cultural workers, healthcare workers, social workers, psychologists and technicians. The interdisciplinary make-up of the team will no doubt have an impact on the rehabilitation delivered. The lack of nurse or clinical psychology support within one team was a subject of criticism, considering that individuals remained at home without any hospital admission (Wolfe et al., 2000). Individual members bring different experiences and have different priorities for rehabilitative input, which can manifest themselves directly into the team approach. Some approaches featured continuous family training, which made having a committed family member to provide ongoing rehabilitation at home obligatory (Pace et al., 1999). Another study used multidisciplinary notes, as well as 'patient-held' records (Rodgers et al., 1997), to promote a more client-directed approach.

Clear arrangements and responsibilities and adequate communication at all levels (between team members themselves, and between team members and their clients and other bodies) are essential for the smooth operation of early discharge schemes (Sims et al., 1997). In the development of community teams the potential benefits of a new style therapist, a generic therapist, have been raised (Barnes, 1994). A generic worker could cross disciplinary boundaries and provide, for example, nursing, social care and support work at one session. This has caused considerable controversy concerning issues of risk and levels of responsibility (Sims et al., 1997; Stevenson, 2000), not to mention the perception of threat to job roles by qualified specialist staff. This is a critical issue and will be addressed in the discussion at the end of the chapter.

Care management

A note about terminology

Quibble over terminology is an ongoing, relentless and necessary procedure in many academic fields. However, at times, agreement to disagree may proffer the best solution. In the event of management of the individual, three terms have been employed interchangeably. They are case management, care management and key working. Rather than trying to tease out the possible similarities and differences between the terms, they will be regarded as one and the same fundamental concept. They differ only in detail. For example, they all represent scenarios in which individual clients are assigned to someone who is responsible for the coordination of their ongoing support, working across different professional borders. This 'support' may vary enormously and this is where the source of difference lies.

Key workers provide the most basic input on this scale. Their role involves coordinating the communication of all those within the immediate environment of their client and this tends to be between the client, his/her family and the team. More often than not key workers are therapists themselves working in acute or postacute settings, but in this role they do not actively provide therapy. Care managers have an added responsibility and are pegged further along the scale. Their work usually revolves predominantly around the needs of their client in the community. The original team providing care may well have disintegrated on discharge from hospital, and it is the role of the care manager to ensure that their clients receive the most appropriate services on offer. This involves knowledge of all the available resources that cross the social and healthcare divide, and more time in which to devote their skills to management rather than any clinical work. Case managers are at the opposite end of the scale. Their job entails organizing their clients' care down to the finest detail, and this will often also include the financial arrangements. Thus while a clinical background is not a necessity, training in managerial skills is a prerequisite for the role.

Due to the conflicting usage of these terms across the literature it will be confusing to retain the preferred term of each individual study. Thus, for the purposes of the next section, the term 'care' manager or 'care' management will be chosen as a generic term to refer to all three. The blurry divisions between their boundaries and the lack of detail in many of the studies was further justification for this action.

The evaluation – care management

In Italy, 200 elderly people already receiving conventional care services were randomly allocated either to an intervention group that provided integrated medical and social care with care management or to a control group that received services as before (Bernabei et al., 1998). The care managers were trainees recruited from a course on care management. After they reported the results of the initial assessment to the geriatric evaluation unit (a geriatrician, a social worker and several nurses), individualized care plans delivered by a multidisciplinary team were made in agreement with GPs. The role of the care manager was to be 'on tap' to deal with any problems, monitor service provision and to guarantee extra help as required by clients and their GPs. While they had a managerial role, it was the GP who held clinical responsibility for each client. For individuals in the care management programme admission to hospital was delayed and less common at 1-year follow-up. They also received less home visits by GPs, increased physical functioning and there was a decrease in the decline of cognitive status. This outcome reduced costs considerably, as compared with the control group who received the conventional and fragmented array of services. Bernabei and colleagues were able to conclude that care management is critical to the success of

community-based programmes whereby it ensures close collaboration between all parties, integrating social and medical care.

A positive outcome was also found in a similar study, whereby elderly individuals with stroke were offered a system of home-based care management
(Goldberg et al., 1997). The treatment team comprised a project physician,
psychologist, recreational therapist and the care manager, who was also a
social worker. The role of the care manager was to address psychosocial
needs, ensure access to information and to identify any problems at an early
stage. This was done via weekly telephone contact and monthly visits and
the assistance and participation of the primary carer was an essential component to the rehabilitation process. It was found that those individuals in
the intervention group were facilitated in general social activities and the
frequency of instrumental activities of daily living increased at 6 months.
However, this difference was not significant at 12 months. Telephone contact was perceived to be as efficacious as in-home visits, thus revealing the
potential for a cheaper alternative.

These two studies have specifically focused on the impact of having a care
manager, and they provide a useful source of evidence for this section. However, alone they do not amount to much. Outcomes from other studies that
incorporate care management into the rehabilitation programme also provide a means for gleaning more information about its effects. Unfortunately,
in most of these studies the details pertaining to the exact role of the care man-
ager/coordinator tend to be limited (Rodgers et al., 1997; Rudd et al., 1997;
Richards et al., 1998; Pace et al., 1999; Wolfe et al., 2000). So, while the outcome may still be, in part, attributable to the presence of a care manager, the
direct influence is unpredictable and it may be unwise to make any inferences
from them. There was one exception, the description of which will follow.

In a pilot study investigating early discharge after stroke, one therapist was
allocated as the care manager using the other therapists on a consultant basis
(Widen Holmqvist et al., 1995). This was not only cost effective by reducing
inpatient admission time, but its participants followed patterns equivalent
to that of other stroke patients. In the trial itself two physical therapists,
two occupational therapists and one speech therapist formed the outreach
team, with a social worker available on a consulting basis (Widen Holmqvist
et al., 1998). Again one therapist was assigned as the care manager for each
client, who acted as the link between hospital and outpatient care. The care

manager was responsible for coordinating the discharge procedure, most of the at-home therapy and the rehabilitation team, and contacting the appropriate neurologist. The outcome was positive (see early-discharge section of multidisciplinary team evaluation) with increased rates of social activity, activities of daily living, motor capacity, manual dexterity and walking. It was also cost-effective.

Discussion

Although the number of studies available to review the efficacy of care-management programmes was few, all found some positive outcomes associated with care-management intervention. Already a lot of heterogeneity can be observed in the structure of each care-management strategy, and this raises questions about their future development. In one study the care managers were recruited directly from a course on care management (Bernabei et al., 1998). Any personal experience in therapeutic rehabilitation was unreported. In another study one of the therapists within the team itself assumed the care managerial role and it varied for each client (Widen Holmqvist et al., 1998). In yet another study there was a specific care manager identified as part of the team, who also happened to be a social worker (Goldberg et al., 1997). Hence these care managers varied at a number of levels such as their professional background, whether they were part of the team, and if they were, whether they provided their own therapeutic input. It would take more detailed analysis to tease out how these factors influence the managerial role and ultimately the outcome.

There may never be agreement regarding the terminology (care/case management/coordination or key working), but it is likely that *what* is provided is more significant than *who* it is provided by. Thus comprehensive job descriptions should be a common feature of future literature in this area. Studies need to be designed in such a way so as to address whether specific training in care management is necessary, or whether it matters what member of a team takes on the role so long as someone does. Even in studies that do not specifically investigate care management, it would be useful if they provided a sufficient description concerning the care-manager role and how it might have impacted on the care provided.

The Northumberland Head Injury Service (NHIS), a community team service in the north of England, provides an example of a care-management system in practice. It sits within a larger care-management network set up across the county. This ensures that any individual with an impairment following an initial hospital admission or a referral from the community itself is each assigned to a care manager (unless they are admitted to a nursing home). Each care manager is part of a local team, supported by a local team manager who is based in a primary care practice. For the NHIS it means that its three (full-time equivalent) care managers, through having access to social services funds, form a bridge between health and social services enabling them to employ a holistic approach to individual client needs. After carrying out an initial assessment, the care manager prioritizes and coordinates interdisciplinary intervention thereafter, involving the carer from the beginning. They pick and choose the most appropriate services for their clients, and monitor their provision, constructing a personalized care-package arrangement. Currently the service actively supports 120 people in their own homes, and remains in lifelong contact with each individual should any needs arise.

The care managers in this particular service come from a variety of professional backgrounds, and are required to complete a 1-day induction training course before they can practice. There is no solid evidence that has confirmed the efficacy of this service. The only evidence lies in observations and feedback, such that families remain together, clients receive their due benefits and that they remain out of hospital.

Individual therapeutic input

Despite the 'togetherness' of modern day rehabilitation, it is important for individual disciplines to assess their techniques. (Rice-Oxley and Turner-Stokes, 1999)

A substantial proportion of the research within the context of community rehabilitation has investigated the efficacy of specific therapeutic input, primarily in the form of occupational therapy and physiotherapy. This may be delivered within a framework of other community services, and possibly by way of a team. Whereby this could have been discussed as part of the multidisciplinary team approach above, these papers do not discuss the team approach as such, but rather the specific impact of individual therapies. Hence this area was considered to warrant individual attention.

Young and Forster (1991, 1992, 1993) have done much work on this subject. In one study they compared day-hospital attendance and at-home physiotherapy for people with stroke after they had been discharged from hospital. The individuals attended the day hospital for 2 days a week or received home treatment from a community physiotherapist; 124 people were recruited and 108 were fully assessed at 6 months. Both arms of the study showed significant improvement in functional abilities between discharge and 6 months but the improvements were significantly greater for those treated at home. This was despite the fact that those treated at home received less actual treatment. Home physiotherapy thus seemed to be somewhat more effective and more resource-efficient than day-hospital attendance and the authors suggested that this should be the preferred long-term method of rehabilitation.

In a similar study design from England, 327 people who were discharged from medical or geriatric wards were randomized into two groups (Gladman et al., 1993; Gladman and Lincoln, 1994). One group received domiciliary rehabilitation at home from physiotherapy, occupational therapy and other relevant professions. The other group received hospital-based rehabilitation in both an outpatient and day-unit setting. At 6 months the outcome was similar for both groups, in terms of functional disability, perceived health, social engagement and life satisfaction. Around 15–20 therapy contacts were required per month within a 6-month time scale to obtain any significant functional benefit.

Elaborate description has been avoided in this evaluation to save the reader from potentially tedious details, however this particular study made some observations that merit further mention. First, in those individuals discharged from a geriatric ward, the hospital-based group had a slightly lower death rate and institutionalization rate than the home-based group. Those discharged from medical wards or the stroke unit showed no difference between the home and hospital-based therapy. This indicates that the location of any acute care received is likely to influence rehabilitation outcome in the long term. The second point was that younger people appeared to have better outcomes within the home, which may not be the case for more elderly clients, indicating that age may also be a confounding factor.

Long-term follow-up rarely favours home therapy outright, but often there are indications that it is preferable. In a 6-week 'domiciliary' intervention programme by an occupational therapist, while activities of daily living were increased at 8 weeks as compared with routine follow-up, this difference was not maintained at 6 months (Gilbertson et al., 2000). However, an increased level of satisfaction was reported in the intervention group at 6 months, and this led to the conclusion that this form of therapy enhanced recovery and reduced deterioration on returning home. Another study helped to maintain individuals at home by providing them with regular reviews from an occupational therapist (Corr and Bayer, 1995). Whilst this did not improve their activities of daily living, the number of readmissions to hospital significantly decreased over a period of 1 year.

There is still controversy over whether such contacts always need to be conducted by qualified therapists. A visit once a week by an occupational and/or physiotherapist who prescribed a programme of exercises and activities for a period of up to 3 months was compared with that of standard outpatient or day-hospital therapy in New Zealand (Baskett et al., 1999). The programme was devised in collaboration with the individual, incorporating goals set towards improving aspects of daily activities in the home beyond that expected by individuals themselves. At 3 months there were no significant differences in neurological, physical and activities of daily living function between the two groups. There were no differences in the number of visits made, but the 'contact time period' for the experimental group was longer, and may have implications for its cost-effectiveness. This study concluded that physical rehabilitation under the regular supervision of qualified therapists but conducted by individuals was as effective as having the individual attend a hospital outpatient department.

It is often thought that delivery of coordinated rehabilitation some time after stroke is not worthwhile as the therapeutic window of rapid recovery in the first few weeks has been missed. This is not necessarily the case. As an example, Werner and Kessler (1996) delivered rehabilitation to 28 people after stroke with 16 controls. These individuals were about 3 years poststroke and were part of an outpatient programme for a total of 12 weeks consisting of an hour of physiotherapy and an hour of occupational therapy five times weekly. The intervention group had clinically relevant functional gains. This also improved self-esteem and reduced levels of depression. Whilst the outcome was positive, the demand for physiotherapy in another study involving the same client group was noted to be small (Green et al., 1999). This was based on current service activity over 1 year and it showed that longer-term poststroke mobility problems can be addressed by a minimum number of three contacts or a treatment period not exceeding 13 weeks. Thus there may be no need for specialist rehabilitation in the presence of a more generic service for people with longer-term stroke-related needs, but intervention of some sort is recommended.

Less common in the literature are studies that have investigated individuals that have not been admitted to hospital following stroke. People who have not spent any time in hospital are less likely to receive community services than those individuals who spend even very short times in hospital (Noad et al., 1998). Research suggests that when this client group does receive occupational therapy input over 5 months, benefits were noted in terms of improved performance of instrumental activities of daily living and a reduced strain on carers (Walker et al., 1999). Such an outcome emphasizes the potential benefits that this client group can experience when often their needs may be ignored. This has important implications for a decreased dependence on social and health resources in the future.

Discussion

Most of the literature that examines the benefit of individual therapeutic input at home is about people who have been admitted to hospital following a stroke. The primary focus of the studies was to investigate the effect of therapy that is delivered to the individual at home immediately following discharge from acute care. Most of these studies have shown this rehabilitation to be if not more effective, at least as effective as routine services (Young and Forster, 1991; Gladman et al., 1993, 1995; Corr and Bayer, 1995; Baskett et al., 1999; Gilbertson, 2000). Where home rehabilitation programmes have been found to be more effective in relation to traditional services, they do not extend across *all* outcome measures (e.g. activities of daily living, client satisfaction, carer strain, cost-effectiveness etc.). Rather, the benefits were usually confined to only one or two variables.

Age, location of hospital admission, length of follow-up and the nature of the control treatment have all influenced the outcome in some way. This has been observed in people with the same diagnosis, at similar times since stroke, receiving similar forms of intervention. However, these findings do not necessarily span the entire population of people with a stroke. Although more specialist rehabilitation may be considered more appropriate for people who have only recently had a stroke, a generic service may be sufficient to meet the needs of people more than 3 years poststroke. For those not admitted to hospital, individual therapeutic intervention may also be appropriate, but it may have different qualities.

Research in this area has spanned the last decade which, for this field, is a relatively long time period. The generally positive results pertaining to provision of home-based therapy has led to it being more widely accepted, paving the way for more specific recommendations (such as the minimum levels required). However, there is still scope for yet more studies to look at the different components of the home rehabilitation programme to identify which may be more or less beneficial than others (Eldar, 2000).

While all these studies have illustrated the effectiveness of home physiotherapy and occupational therapy services, these are not necessarily in isolation. Many of the people in these studies will have been receiving support from a number of other community services, and thus the benefits may not be entirely attributed to that specific intervention. It is realized that individual community therapists need to be part of a specialist stroke team, be correctly resourced, integrated into primary-care services and have strong links with social services and voluntary organizations (Gilbertson, 2000). Where this specifically referred to occupational therapists, no doubt it also applies for other individual therapists. Thus there may be use in investigating the individual impact of each therapy for research, but in reality a single therapeutic intervention may not be appropriate. It was disappointing to note that in both arms of one study more than a third of people were depressed at some point and a quarter of carers were emotionally distressed (Young and Forster, 1991, 1992). This serves to reinforce the notion that any home rehabilitation programme needs to address the psychosocial needs as well as the physical needs of both the person with stroke and the family.

Researching the benefits of single therapeutic disciplines does not necessitate a stroke population, it just happens that this is where the literature circulates. As well as there being a lack of evidence for those people with other diagnoses, the literature is sparse in relation to the efficacy of other disciplines. Therefore, more studies are required that focus on intervention by other single disciplines (such as speech and language therapy, clinical psychology and perhaps dietary advice), and with a wider range of individuals with different impairments.

Nursing intervention

Nurse practitioners have been evaluated as primary-care providers for more than 25 years (Mundinger et al., 2000) but there is a shortage of large-scale, randomized design trials that compare nurse practitioners with physicians. A meta-analysis of 38 studies indicated a trend to suggest that nurse practitioner care is equivalent to or sometimes better than care provided by a physician (Brown and Grimes, 1995). Patient compliance was found to be significantly higher for individuals seen by nurse practitioners. However, as well as lacking methodological rigour, these studies were designed around the care provider, reporting little about the care process itself. The activities of the care provider could therefore not be related to any of the outcomes, nor was there sufficient evidence to monitor cost-effectiveness.

A recent study was able to overcome some of these methodological flaws (Mundinger et al., 2000). Of 3397 adults screened at five primary care clinics following an emergency department or urgent care visit, 1997 people were recruited and randomized to either a nurse practitioner or physician. Of these, 1316 people kept their initial primary care appointments and were subsequently enrolled; diagnoses included diabetes, asthma and hypertension. Each individual then became a part of their newly appointed practice sites, and the care provider assigned to them managed any further treatment. The primary-care nurse practitioners and physicians did not vary in the type of clients that they were assigned to, and they shared similar responsibilities in terms of their authority to prescribe, consult, refer and admit patients. Furthermore, they drew from the same pool of specialists, inpatient units and emergency departments. At 1 year after the initial appointment, the study concluded that in ambulatory care situations patient outcomes (e.g. self-reported health status, patient satisfaction, health service utilization and physiological measures) were comparable. There were minor statistical differences on particular subscales but these were unlikely to be of any real clinical significance.

While this study is of interest in terms of confirming the effectiveness of nurse practitioners in a primary healthcare setting, only a small proportion of the client population had neurological impairments and thus it may not be generalizable to this group as a whole. It also reveals nothing about the feasibility of delivering nursing intervention to individuals in their home.

A study by Forster and Young (1996) was able to go some way to remedy this situation. They randomly assigned 240 elderly individuals who had recently had a stroke and were living at home to an intervention group or a control group. Both groups received the usual treatment and services provided by hospital and community staff, but only the intervention group received additional visits by a specialist outreach nurse over a period of 12 months. A minimum of six visits in the first 6 months by a specialist outreach nurse was shown to be as effective as the standard treatment in terms of perceived health, social activities and stress among carers. For mildly disabled individuals intervention elicited benefits in the form of a small increase in social activities. Although this quantitative report which focused on the psychosocial aspects of stroke rehabilitation was unable to distinguish any major benefits of specialist nurse input, qualitative analysis proved to be more illuminating. It concluded that a 'valued, flexible, individualised service had been provided' (Dowswell et al., 1997). Personalized support, practical help, information, interest and counselling were the factors noted to be of particular value to clients.

Comparable outcomes were also noted in a study that compared a home programme of rehabilitation for individuals with moderately severe traumatic brain injury against a standard inpatient programme (Warden et al., 2000). Further analysis showed that less severely injured people tended to do better when treated at home, whereas the more severely injured individuals did better in the hospital programme. Although this study did not specifically investigate the singular impact of nurse intervention, a nurse was at the core of the study design. Following an initial 5-day multidisciplinary evaluation and medical treatment as appropriate, a psychiatric nurse provided guidance on home activities, as well as making weekly telephone calls, as part of an 8-week home programme. Not only was this shown to be a viable treatment option, it provided effective care at a lower cost than inpatient care.

Discussion

While one trial investigated the impact of nurse intervention in *addition* to other standard treatment (Forster and Young, 1996; Dowswell et al., 1997), another study drew a comparison between nurse and physician care (Mundinger et al., 2000). Comparable outcomes were found in most studies, which questions the way in which nursing care should ideally be delivered.

If rehabilitation is found to be as effective with specialist nurse outreach as without it, then justifying it as an additional service may be difficult. It may be that it will only be cost-effective for those receiving little or no support. This has implications for the establishment of a more generic community rehabilitation worker. An investigation into the contribution of nursing to an interprofessional community-based rehabilitation team documented the importance of their interpersonal and information-giving skills (Shiu et al., 1999). However, there were difficulties in trying to distinguish nursing contribution from that of other health professionals. While the authors noted a need for nurses as well as other health professionals, the observed overlap of roles within a team may be a further indication that a generic team worker can provide a similar service, and simultaneously cut costs.

Specialist outreach

The primary goal of outreach programmes is to provide rural communities with rehabilitation services that would otherwise only be available in urban institutions. (Sullivan et al., personal communication)

Organizing locally based comprehensive rehabilitation services in rural areas has been met with success (Lazarus et al., 1984). However, the literature usually comprises descriptions of programmes, rather than actual evidence to evaluate their efficacy. Following an overview in this field by Flynn and Volpe (1993), Wilson and colleagues (1995) responded to the recommendation that quality of care should be integral to any evaluative efforts. Levels of customer satisfaction were thus examined for those utilizing a mobile clinic that provides consultation services in 15 rural communities in eastern and northeastern Ontario, Canada (Wilson et al., 1995). The mobile clinic consists of an interdisciplinary team of professionals that includes a physician, a nurse, a physiotherapist, a speech and language therapist, an occupational therapist, a social worker, a psychologist, a secretary, a driver and other specialists if necessary. Team members are made available as required; one of whom assumes the coordinating role. It was found that 147 out of 168 surveys sent out were completed and 97.2% of respondents stated that they preferred to be seen in their own communities by the mobile clinic. Enhanced accessibility was regarded as the major advantage. Despite this high satisfaction rate there were several critical comments pertaining to procedural and communicative issues, the perception of no practical benefits and insufficient visits. The primary concern, however, seemed to be the absence of any assured continuity of care by the clinic, and the subsequent dependency on local healthcare workers to manage ongoing care. Clients, after all, remain the responsibility of the local workers. The role of the clinic may therefore be more about establishing individual rehabilitation programmes and training community health workers, rather than providing practical care itself. Hence it would share many of the principles of community-based rehabilitation projects in the South (see Chapter 8).

At a different level (due to the relatively shorter distances involved), outreach programmes have also been examined in the UK. This takes the form of specialist care being provided in general practices as opposed to in hospitals. Reduced travelling times and more convenience were seen to be the benefits of specialist outreach clinics in general practice (Bailey et al., 1994) as perceived by the professionals themselves. Along with a reduction in waiting times, this has contributed to a rapid growth in this form of provision. However, despite their location, there is still little interaction between specialists and GPs, which may decrease resource efficiency. Investigation regarding the opinions of the public regarding this service has yet to be formally reviewed, especially with regards to neurological rehabilitation.

Chandler et al. (personal communication) found that in a review of community services in northeast England there was inequity of both service provision and its accessibility. For an individual with a neurological impairment, service provision depends upon their geographical location, diagnosis and age. One recommendation stated that there should be no longer than 1 hour of travel time involved in the delivery of rehabilitation services. In this particular locality this was made possible by forming two satellite clinics in strategically placed centres. These new centres were also hoped to form the base from which further good practice could grow.

Discussion

Unsurprisingly, outreach is more a feature of rehabilitation programmes in countries where there are large expanses of rural land, such as the USA, Canada and Australia. Outreach programmes still have a role in more densely populated areas such as the UK but they are more likely to be 'institution-based', as opposed to 'network systems' (as classified in Sullivan et al., personal communication). Where the former typically consists of rehabilitation specialists from institutions travelling to rural communities, the latter function by coordinating the delivery of specialized rehabilitation services to regional communities. The literature seems to illuminate the benefits of outreach but raises questions as to its purpose. This may be found best applied to training and development, rather than practical clinical advice. An increase in communication between the outreach body and the local healthcare workers or GP may also serve to maximize the benefits of outreach.

Other aspects of community rehabilitation

Three other studies stood out in the literature that failed to find a home within the previous sections. They are described in this section as they represent unique investigations into aspects of community rehabilitation that may inspire more studies to come. The first examined the role of a referrals facilitator between primary care and the voluntary sector, and it was shown to result in clinically important benefits compared with standard GP care (Grant et al., 2000). It reduced anxiety and improved ability to carry out everyday activities and feelings about general health and quality of life. However, it was at a greater expense, especially considering that it did not save time in primary care. Links between the statutory services and voluntary care are renowned for being poor, remaining as largely discrete service bodies. Despite the increasing cost, long-term implications of a better referral system to voluntary agencies may well have positive consequences.

The second study describes a hospital discharge scheme for the elderly using care attendants to accompany individuals home on the first day and provide up to 12 hours of support a week for 2 weeks (Townsend et al., 1988). It was shown to decrease hospital readmission rates. There were no significant differences between the two groups (the control group received standard aftercare) in physical independence, morale or in death rates. In this study the care attendants provided practical care, encouraged individuals to do things on their own, and organized help from family, friends and statutory services.

The third study compared a residential postacute rehabilitation programme for people with traumatic brain injury with that of standard home-based services (Willer et al., 1999). This study is of interest for two reasons. First, the residential programme incorporated care-coordinated rehabilitation. Second, it was unlike other contemporary studies, because the participants allocated to home-based rehabilitation represented the control group. This group received variable service provision, while the individuals in the residential programme received intensive care-coordinated rehabilitation. Results indicated that those people in the residential programme displayed a statistically significant increase in functional abilities, specifically relating to motor skills and cognitive ability. The care-coordinated support provided by a neuropsychologist may have been a key factor in the success of the residential programme. Even though the control group made less significant improvements, of particular interest was that they had a superior level of community integration at the beginning of the study and maintained this high level throughout follow-up. This may be significant for the future of home-based services.

Discussion

The first two studies highlighted discrete investigations about the rehabilitation process whereby additional intervention may prove to be a vital contributing factor in prolonging the effects of rehabilitation. Being single study areas, more research would be required to implement them widely into practice, but they are promising initiatives for the future of rehabilitation in the community. If community integration positively correlates with an increased quality of life then the findings from the third study may be crucial in promoting the home as the rehabilitation setting of the future.

Overview of the evidence base for community rehabilitation

Most of the studies reviewed in this chapter have indicated that community rehabilitation, in whatever form (e.g. via a team, individual intervention, care-managed or as an outreach programme), is at least as effective as the traditional alternatives (e.g. hospital care, day care, residential care or outpatient services). However, it is important to be aware that even with sufficient evidence to support that rehabilitation in the home is effective, it does not necessarily mean that people want it (Neuberger, 1992). While the evidence is very promising at a glance, these papers range enormously in their aims, and thus comprehensive and thorough grounding to support a particular intervention is rare. Nevertheless, together they provide some valuable information about rehabilitative research for the future and how it should be applied to the stark reality of living in the community.

This overview will not entail further discussion pertaining to the efficacy of any individual studies unless specifically relevant (for this information refer to the individual discussion sections throughout the chapter). Rather this section aims to summarize the main themes of the chapter and conclude with some recommendations for the future. Stroke is the most investigated area of neurological rehabilitation to date and thus, to begin this section, it will be used to paint a portrait of developments so far and put rehabilitation research into perspective.

Stroke rehabilitation

Neurological rehabilitation research has largely focused on the stroke population, with over 800 randomized controlled trials in stroke research, and five new trials being identified every week (Rice-Oxley and Turner-Stokes, 1999). This is in accordance with the overwhelming majority of studies reported in this chapter that have investigated individuals who have experienced a stroke. A recent review of services for helping acute stroke patients to avoid hospital admission concluded that there was no evidence to support a radical shift in the care of acute stroke patients from hospital-based care (Langhorne et al., 2000). Where hospital inpatient admission may seem to be the best option during the acute phase of stroke this stay may be reduced by effective rehabilitation provided in the community in all phases of stroke (Eldar, 2000). In most of the postacute rehabilitation literature, follow-up and links with community are seen to be essential to maintain and further benefits (Hawley et al., 2000).

Despite these encouraging findings, the picture of stroke rehabilitation is still not complete. Even within the same client population, the trials in this review were characterized by considerable heterogeneity, making it difficult to draw specific conclusions. This suggests that there are still an insufficient number of studies in the literature to make any solid conclusions. Bearing in mind the relatively large amount of studies that have already investigated stroke rehabilitation, there appears to be a long way to go before we can expect to have enough literature to fully support any particular practice. This point is emphasized in a review of stroke care in Europe revealing that there was no standardized format with which to compare the data available from each country, and the data from some countries (e.g. Spain and Hungary) were very sparse indeed (Wolfe et al., 1995).

Less press, smaller numbers and further heterogeneity among the head-injured population confound the use of randomized controlled trials but this does not negate their need for good management (Rice-Oxley and Turner-Stokes, 1999). This will also be true of many other client populations in the neurological sphere. This is because although strokes, head injuries and multiple sclerosis account for the majority of people with neurological impairments there is an enormous number of rarer diagnoses; diagnoses that will not even get a mention in the literature. Put into perspective, this creates rather a dim portrait of the state of community rehabilitation research today, but there may be other reasons why our understanding in this area is insufficient. One of these reasons may be associated with methodological design.

Methodological design

Despite not having enough studies per se, the differences within each study design make it inherently difficult to compare and contrast their findings. Variations in the measures used, participant demographics, diagnosis and criteria for entry into the study impact on the outcome in unique ways. However, the most common criticism of the studies reviewed was that their sample sizes were insufficient so as to confirm statistical significance. They may provide some illuminating observations but without statistical significance their use is of little value in scientific circles.

In one study patient suitability required that a 'positive rehabilitative outcome' was to be expected (Richards et al., 1998), which may not be fairly compared with a study where participants are not attributed with the same potential. Other factors that alter clinical outcomes are the differences in lengths of intervention and the intensity of therapy provided. Randomized controlled trials differ from more evaluative before and after designs, making comparative conclusions not viable. Some studies carry out in-depth cost analyses and include follow-up trials, whereas others have alternative foci with more qualitative leanings. All these factors contribute to the already difficult task of evaluating this study area.

Assessment

The measures that assess outcomes are fundamental to the value of a study. Many of the more commonly used outcome measures assess specific aspects of functional ability, which take little account of living conditions and quality of life. There is a notable lack of standardized home-based assessments (Pace et al., 1999), which makes it difficult to design studies that accurately convey the effectiveness of rehabilitation in a community setting, especially with regards to quality of life. One could argue that components of consumer satisfaction should be investigated as a priority over clinical variables. Clinical outcome may vary tremendously, but if a client is satisfied with the service provided and his/her own rehabilitative process, then it could be argued that the ultimate outcome has been reached. If the assessment measure is not adequately reflecting a client's view then that is another matter for debate. If clients are accurately informed at the outset of intervention as to its aims and scope, then it is likely that a realistic expectation will have been met and they may be subsequently highly satisfied. This throws the value of a satisfaction rating into jeopardy. While there are no answers at this stage it is clear that more investigation is required to develop more sensitive measures that assess the critical factors of recovery. These factors may not necessarily be viewed in the same way (i.e. clients and providers may have different ideas about the same care), and this must be taken into consideration.

The discrepancy between professional and client perspectives was highlighted in a study about the reliability of client reports. Comparisons were made between the reports of 124 individuals with stroke not admitted to hospital with that of the service providers about the rehabilitation services delivered (Luther et al., 1998). Hospital services, social services and community services were all investigated and it was concluded that the reports did not always tally. There was some indication that those people with greater impairments and those with perceptual problems were more likely to disagree. Departmental records may also have been inaccurate. Clearly this result stresses that care should be taken in interpreting any information about service provision from any source.

Individual needs and perception

On a macroscopic scale, there may be some very obvious differences in the rehabilitative needs across various diagnostic categories, i.e. people with the same diagnosis will share the same general needs. However, these tend to be very crudely defined and of little value. Analysis at a more detailed level reveals that even when individuals have the same diagnosis, each has complex and unique needs that change over time. The literature is full of endless observations indicating that factors such as diagnosis, age, severity of impairment and geographical location all influence the demand and efficacy of rehabilitation services. This is in addition to the contribution of spontaneous recovery. Thus, in developing rehabilitation in the community we need to take this on board and aim to provide adaptable services that can accommodate for such an unpredictable demand.

It is not only need itself that varies, but also individual perceptions of needs and impairments in general. It was shown in one study that initial perceptions of illness were an important determinant of recovery after myocardial infarction (Petrie et al., 1996). If the illness was perceived to last a short time then this was a significant predictor of return to work within 6 weeks. Attendance on the rehabilitation course was significantly related to a stronger belief during admission that the illness could be cured or controlled. This finding could provide the basis for predicting outcomes, and thus ways to encourage positive perceptions may be a challenge for the future.

Applicability

An important aspect of research is the applicability of study findings to the real world. An elaborate study that makes lengthy conclusions that cannot be replicated outside of test conditions has only limited value. This was raised in one particular study (Bernabei et al., 1998) but is likely to be the case in many more. In this instance, even though a hospital at home programme was found to be cost-effective they were hesitant about it remaining that way when delivered as a standard service in the community. They noted that the advent of a new community service may attract all sorts of customers that would otherwise not have bothered to seek help at all, or would have found an alternative.

Generic working or skillblending

The presence of some form of generic worker involved in the provision of rehabilitation in the community has been raised on a number of occasions in this chapter. The primary reason for this is that there are usually insufficient resources to support a large range of qualified therapists. Another perhaps more pertinent reason is that when people do have access to a variety of professional expertise there tends to be overlap. This causes not only confusion on the part of the client and family, but conflict between professionals themselves.

Barnes (1994) noted a preference for the term 'rehabilitation therapist' as opposed to a 'generic therapist'. This then expels the illusion of having created a 'jack of all trades and a master of none'. He envisaged their training to be geared towards that of client groups (i.e. children, the elderly, people with learning and mental health impairments) rather than through therapy professions. These individuals would then be responsible for the majority of the case load but specialist referral would be deemed necessary for a minority, much as is the case for GP practices in the UK today.

There are obvious advantages for a generic practitioner. As well as making it less confusing for the client, it would be less time consuming, and less overlap would mean greater cost returns in the long term. The problems that arise through miscommunication and bad coordination within team management would not arise and individuals would be more likely to get, and have greater access to, support.

However, these benefits do not come without their drawbacks. In a study of staff perspectives of a hospital at home scheme, 'healthcare support workers' under the supervision of and in consultation with health professionals assisted in the delivery of care (Sims et al., 1997). Their tasks included washing and dressing the client, and helping with household tasks; a role that combined elements of nursing, social care and therapy. Some staff reported being anxious about the responsibilities taken on by these individuals. This may also be the case for a rehabilitation therapist. A rehabilitation therapist network would require a radical change to the system which would incur high initial costs for the implementation of new training programmes. This could be construed as a relatively cheap alternative in the long run, but at the expense of quality. There is also the possibility that such personnel are perceived to be a threat to qualified staff in terms of their individual jobs and their profession as a whole (Gibbs et al., 1991). However, our duty is to our disabled clients, and if there are more effective alternatives we should study these options.

Perhaps a rehabilitation therapist is not the solution to finding more effective rehabilitation. Laidler (1994) acknowledges that multidisciplinary teamwork is effective and that the client should always be at the centre of the care network. Due to either a lack of interdisciplinary working or in contrast, too much duplication, clients have not always received the holistic care they require. Laidler proposes the concept of 'skillblending'. She defines this as 'an inter-professional relationship in which the work of each professional is supported by – and in turn supports and reinforces – the work of others' (Laidler, 1994). The necessity for individual expertise within a team structure is reinforced, but the interdisciplinary working is regarded as being integral to effective rehabilitation.

It may be that both skillblending and rehabilitation therapists have a part to play in the future but at different points in the rehabilitation process. A more generic therapist may be more appropriate for clients with long-term needs, whereas skillblending may be better applied to acute and postacute settings. Both are promising avenues to explore, but without further investigation of these resourceful initiatives their potential will remain untapped.

The future

Not only do there need to be more studies per se, but also these studies need to be of a high quality. This includes having an extensive range of valid measurement techniques and materials and a trial design that evaluates community intervention in relation to the best available alternative. They need also to be designed to answer worthwhile questions. For example, instead of just comparing a care-management service with that of standard service provision, investigations need to probe deeper. Variations in the quality of service provision may be due to specific individuals involved. Thus a study design to compare care-management schemes which are headed by care managers from different backgrounds may prove to be more insightful. This could inform care-management training programmes so that the success of a service can be imputed to the care-management system and not a particular individual. This would then have a wider impact on the world of rehabilitation.

This chapter has reviewed the literature that provides evidence about the efficacy of community rehabilitation. This has been largely restricted to rehabilitation that is only delivered at home or in the community itself. While this was a necessary parameter of the review it does not illuminate the benefits of community rehabilitation when it works in close conjunction with institutions and hospital wards. There are many recommendations for a closer integration of hospital and community services. Around 90% of people were perceived to have maintained or improved their social and psychological status after being registered with such a service (Roy, 1991). It seems that rather than trying to *compare* the efficacy of rehabilitation in the community with that delivered in hospital, thereby creating a competitive agenda, it may be more useful to focus on how to better address methods of integration to facilitate a smooth continuity of care.

Factors of integration need to be addressed across the board, not only between hospital and community, but also with primary care. General practitioners often have clinical responsibility for many people who also require rehabilitation services but communication between various health professionals is virtually absent. In the example of the mobile outreach team in Canada (Wilson et al., 1995), the connections between the mobile team and the local health workers were perceived to be integral to its future success and the satisfaction of its clients. The programme could then be designed in such a way so as to facilitate better communication, increasing its resource efficiency. It is apparent that the increase in workload of primary healthcare workers must be alleviated in some way.

There are many successful projects and services across the globe, but without the skills and funding to disseminate their knowledge, their secrets remain untapped. They provide the ideal opportunity to further our understanding. In the meantime, no doubt, the constant production of studies will continue and hopefully this will provide further insight. Perhaps the only conclusion to make at this point is that with a positive outcome being such a subjective phenomenon, it may be more helpful to investigate the benefits of rehabilitation from the client perspective; an area largely neglected in current research today.

Conclusion

Considering the relatively short life of rehabilitation research the great breadth of the findings must be applauded. However, in relation to what is required, the future of this research will be long and challenging. For community rehabilitation to be taken seriously as a viable alternative or addition to rehabilitation services, not only is there need of a larger number of studies, but high methodological quality is paramount within such a diverse client group. Greater detail is required to identify the critical factors that determine efficacy. When consistently high-quality research is being generated in large amounts it will be possible to make more informed recommendations concerning rehabilitation techniques in the future.

Postscript

After preparation of this book a further valuable randomized controlled trial of community-based rehabilitation after severe traumatic brain injury has been published (Powell et al., 2002). This study compared outreach treatment (mean of two sessions per week for around 27 weeks) in community settings, such as homes, day centres and work places with provision of written information detailing alternative resources. Follow-up for around 2 years was carried out by a blinded independent assessor. All participants had sustained severe traumatic brain injury between 3 months and 20 years previously. A total of 110 individuals were initially allocated to the study, with 48 in the outreach group and 46 in the information group. The primary outcome measures were the Barthel index and the Brain Injury Community Rehabilitation Outcome – 39 (BICRO–39). Secondary measures were the Functional Independence Measure and the Functional Assessment Measure (FIM and FAM) as well as the Hospital Anxiety and Depression Scale. Outreach participants are significantly more likely to shown gains on the Barthel index and the BICRO–39 total score. There were also improvements on the FIM/FAM for personal care and cognitive functions. This study suggested that even years after injury an active community rehabilitation programme can yield benefits and that such benefits may even outlive the active treatment period.

REFERENCES

Bailey, J.J., Black, M.E. and Wilkin, D. (1994). Specialist outreach clinics in general practice. *British Medical Journal* **308**, 1083–6.

Barnes, M.P. (1994). A new style therapist for the real world. *Therapy Weekly* **20**, 47.

Baskett, J.J., Broad, J.B., Reekie, G. et al. (1999). Shared responsibility for ongoing rehabilitation: a new approach to home-based therapy after stroke. *Clinical Rehabilitation* **13**, 23–33.

Beech, R., Rudd, A.G., Tilling, K. and Wolfe, C.D.A. (1999). Economic consequences of early inpatient discharge to community based rehabilitation for stroke in an inner-London teaching hospital. *Stroke* **30**, 729–35.

Bernabei, R., Landi, F., Gambassi, G. et al. (1998). Randomised trial of impact of model of integrated care and case management for older people living in the community. *British Medical Journal* **316**, 1348–51.

Brown, S.A. and Grimes, D.E. (1995). A meta-analysis of nurse practitioners and nurse midwives in primary care. *Nursing Research* **44**, 332–9.

Coast, J., Richards, H.R., Peters, T.J. et al. (1998). Hospital at home or acute hospital care? A cost minimisation analysis. *British Medical Journal* **316**, 1802–6.

Corr, S. and Bayer, A. (1995). Occupational therapy for stroke patients after hospital discharge – a randomised controlled trial. *Clinical Rehabilitation* **9**, 291–6.

Dowswell, G., Lawler, J., Young, J. et al. (1997). A qualitative study of specialist nurse support for stroke patients and care-givers at home. *Clinical Rehabilitation* **11**, 293–301.

Eldar, R. (2000). Rehabilitation in the community for patients with stroke: a review. *Topics in Stroke Rehabilitation* **6**, 48–59.

Flynn, R.J. and Volpe, R. (1993). Issues and choices in the evaluation of out-reach rehabilitation programs. *Canadian Journal of Rehabilitation* **6**, 266–80.

Forster, A. and Young, J. (1996). Specialist nurse support for patients with stroke in the community: a randomised controlled trial. *British Medical Journal* **312**, 1642–6.

Gibbs, I., McCaughan, D. and Griffiths, M. (1991). Skill mix in nursing: a selective review of the literature. *Journal of Advanced Nursing* **16**, 242–9.

Gilbertson, L. (2000). Home rehab improves stroke outcomes. *Health and Ageing* (May), 49–51.

Gilbertson, L., Langhorne, P., Walker, A. et al. (2000). Domiciliary occupational therapy for patients with stroke discharged from hospital: randomised controlled trial. *British Medical Journal* **320**, 603–6.

Gladman, J.R.F. and Lincoln, N.B. (1994). Follow-up of a controlled trial of domiciliary stroke rehabilitation (DOMINO Study). *Age and Ageing* **23**, 9–13.

Gladman, J.R.F., Lincoln, N.B. and Barer, D.H. (1993). A randomised controlled trial of domiciliary and hospital-based rehabilitation for stroke patients after discharge from hospital. *Journal of Neurology, Neurosurgery and Psychiatry* **56**, 960–6.

Gladman, J.R.F., Juby, L.C., Clarke, P.A. et al. (1995). Survey of a domiciliary stroke rehabilitation service. *Clinical Rehabilitation* **9**, 245–9.

Goldberg, G., Segal, M.E., Berk, S.N. et al. (1997). Stroke transition after inpatient rehabilitation. *Topics in Stroke Rehabilitation* **4**, 64–79.

Grant, C., Goodenough, T., Harvey, I. and Hine, C. (2000). A randomised controlled trial and economic evaluation of a referrals facilitator between primary care and the voluntary sector. *British Medical Journal* **320**, 419–23.

Green, J., Forster, A. and Young, J. (1999). A survey of community physiotherapy provision after 1 year post-stroke. *British Journal of Therapy and Rehabilitation* **6**, 216–21.

Hakuno, A., Ito, T., Koike, J. et al. (1996). Home rehabilitation project for home-bound physically disabled people in Yokohama. *Clinical Rehabilitation* **10**, 283–7.

Hawley, C., Stilwell, J., Davies, C. and Stilwell, P. (2000). Post-acute rehabilitation after traumatic brain injury. *British Journal of Therapy and Rehabilitation* **7**, 116–22.

Hensher, M., Fulop, N., Hood, S. and Ujah, S. (1996). Does hospital-at-home make economic sense? Early discharge versus standard care for orthopaedic patients. *Journal of the Royal Society of Medicine* **89**, 548–51.

Iliffe, S. (1998). Hospital at home: from red to amber: data that will reassure advocated – but without satisfying the sceptics. *British Medical Journal* **316**, 1761–2.

Jones, A.L., Charlesworth, J.F. and Hendra, T.J. (2000). Patient mood and carer strain during stroke rehabilitation in the community following early hospital discharge. *Disability and Rehabilitation* **22**, 490–4.

Lafferty, G. (1996). Community based alternatives to hospital rehabilitation services: a review of the evidence and suggestions for approaching future evaluations. *Review of Clinical Gerontology* **6**, 183–94.

Laidler, P. (1994). *Stroke Rehabilitation – Structure and Strategy*. London: Chapman and Hall.

Langhorne, P., Dennis, M.S., Kalra, L. et al. (2000). Services for helping acute stroke patients avoid hospital admission [Review]. *The Cochrane Database of Systematic Reviews* (Issue 2). The Cochrane Library.

Lazarus, S.S., Page, C. and Barcome, D.F. (1984). Rehabilitation services in rural communities: delivery by hospital based and local teams. *Archives of Physical Medicine and Rehabilitation* **65**, 383–7.

Luther, A., Lincoln, N.B. and Grant, F. (1998). Reliability of stroke patients' reports on rehabilitation services received. *Clinical Rehabilitation* **12**, 238–44.

McNamee, P., Christensen, J., Soutter, J. et al. (1998). Cost analysis of early supported hospital discharge for stroke. *Age and Ageing* **27**, 345–51.

Mundinger, M.O., Kane, R.L., Lenz, E.R. et al. (2000). Primary care outcomes in patients treated by nurse practitioners or physicians. *Journal of the American Medical Association* **283**, 59–68.

Neuberger, J. (1992). *Patients' perspectives. From hospital to home care: the potential for acute service provision in the home.* Wales: Welsh Health Planning Forum; The NHS in Wales World Health Organisation; Regional Office for Europe, King's Fund Centre.

Noad, R., Lincoln, N.B. and Challen, K. (1998). Community and hospital stroke patients: long term rehabilitation. *British Journal of Therapy and Rehabilitation* **5**, 578–81.

Pace, G.M., Schlund, M.W., Hazard-Haupt, T. et al. (1999). Characteristics and outcomes of a home and community-based neurorehabilitation programme. *Brain Injury* **13**, 535–46.

Petrie, K.J., Weinman, J., Sharpe, N. and Buckley, J. (1996). Role of patients' view of their illness in predicting return to work and functioning after myocardial infarction: longitudinal study. *British Medical Journal* **312**, 1191–4.

Plant, R., Tait, B., Dawson, P. and Buri, H. (2000). *Community Stroke Rehabilitation Team Evaluation Project: Executive Summary*. Newcastle upon Tyne: Institute of Rehabilitation.

Powell, J., Heslin, J. and Greenwood, R. (2002). Community based rehabilitation after severe traumatic brain injury: a randomised controlled trial. *Journal of Neurology, Neurosurgery and Psychiatry* **72**, 193–202.

Pozzilli, C., Pisani, A., Palmisano, L. et al. (1999). Service location in multiple sclerosis: home or hospital. In *Advances in Multiple Sclerosis: Clinical Research and Therapy*, ed. S. Fredrickson and H. Link, pp. 173–80. London: Martin Dunitz.

Rice-Oxley, M. and Turner-Stokes, L. (1999). Effectiveness of brain injury rehabilitation. *Clinical Rehabilitation* **13** (Suppl. 1), 7–24.

Richards, S.H., Coast, J., Gunnell, D.J. et al. (1998). Randomised controlled trial comparing effectiveness and acceptability of an early discharge, hospital at home scheme with acute hospital care. *British Medical Journal* **316**, 1796–801.

Rodgers, H., Soutter, J., Kaiser, W. et al. (1997). Early supported hospital discharge following acute stroke: pilot study results. *Clinical Rehabilitation* **11**, 280–7.

Roy, C.W. (1991). An integrated community and hospital service for adults with physical disability: 2 years experience. *New Zealand Medical Journal* **104**, 382–4.

Rudd, A.G., Wolfe, C.D.A., Tilling, K. and Beech, R. (1997). "Randomised controlled trial to evaluate early discharge scheme for patients with stroke." *British Medical Journal* **315**, 1039–44.

Shepperd, S. and Iliffe, S. (2000). Hospital at home versus inpatient hospital care [Review]. *The Cochrane Database of Systematic Reviews.* (Issue 2). The Cochrane Library.

Shiu, A.T.Y., Twinn, S.F. and Holroyd, E. (1999). The contribution of nursing to an interprofessional community-based rehabilitation team: perceptions of nurses, patients and carers. *Journal of Interprofessional Care* **13**, 65–75.

Sims, J., Rink, E., Walker, R. and Pickard, L. (1997). The introduction of a hospital at home service: a staff perspective. *Journal of Interprofessional Care* **11**, 217–24.

Stevenson, D. (2000). Rehabilitation outreach: a grounded theory study. *British Journal of Therapy and Rehabilitation* **7**, 112–15.

Townsend, J., Piper, M., Frank, A.O. et al. (1988). Reduction in hospital readmission stay of elderly patients by a community based hospital discharge scheme: a randomised controlled trial. *British Medical Journal* **297**, 544–7.

von Koch, L., Widen Holmqvist, L., Kostulas, V. et al. (2000). A randomised controlled trial of rehabilitation at home after stroke in southwest Stockholm: outcome at six months. *Scandinavian Journal of Rehabilitation Medicine* **32**, 80–6.

Wade, D.T., Langton-Hewer, R., Skilbeck, C.E. et al. (1985). Controlled trial of a home-care service for acute stroke patients. *Lancet* **1**, 323–6.

Walker, M.F., Gladman, J.R.F., Lincoln, N.B. et al. (1999). Occupational therapy for stroke patients not admitted to hospital: a randomised controlled trial. *Lancet* **354**, 278–80.

Warden, D.L., Salazar, A., Martin, E.M. et al. (2000). A home program of rehabilitation for moderately severe traumatic brain injury patients. *Journal of Head Trauma Rehabilitation* **15**, 1092–102.

Werner, R.A. and Kessler, S. (1996). Effectiveness of an intensive outpatient rehabilitation programmed for post acute stroke patients. *American Journal of Physical Medicine and Rehabilitation* **75**, 114–20.

Widen Holmqvist, L., de Pedro-Cuest, J., Holm, M. and Kostulas, V. (1995). Intervention design for rehabilitation at home after stroke: a pilot feasibility study. *Scandinavian Journal of Rehabilitation Medicine* **27**, 43–50.

Widen Holmqvist, L., von Koch, L., Kostulas, V. et al. (1998). A randomised controlled trial of rehabilitation at home after stroke in southwest Stockholm. *Stroke* **29**, 591–7.

Widen Holmqvist, L., von Koch, L. and de Pedro-Cuesta, J. (2000). Use of healthcare, impact on family caregivers and patient satisfaction of rehabilitation at home after stroke in southwest Stockholm. *Scandinavian Journal of Rehabilitation Medicine* **32**, 173–9.

Willer, B., Button, J. and Rempel, R. (1999). Residential and home-based postacute rehabilitation of individuals with traumatic brain injury: a case control study. *Archives of Physical Medicine and Rehabilitation* **80**, 399–404.

Wilson, A., Wynn, A. and Bergstrom, J. (1997). Hospital at home: the use of a new service. *British Journal of Community Health Nursing* **2**, 234–7.

Wilson, A., Parker, H., Wynn, A. et al. (1999). Randomised controlled trial of effectiveness of Leicester hospital at home scheme compared with hospital care. *British Medical Journal* **319**, 1542–6.

Wilson, K.G., Crupi, C.D., Greene, G. et al. (1995). Consumer satisfaction with a rehabilitation mobile outreach program. *Archives of Physical Medicine and Rehabilitation* **76**, 899–904.

Wolfe, C.D.A., Beech, R., Ratcliffe, M. and Rudd, A.G. (1995). Stroke care in Europe: can we learn lessons from the different ways stroke is managed in different countries? *Journal of the Royal Society of Health* **115**, 143–7.

Wolfe, C., Rudd, A. and Tilling, K. (1998). Trials of community rehabilitation need to be of adequate sample size. *Stroke* **29**, 1737–9.

Wolfe, C.D.A., Tilling, K. and Rudd, A.G. (2000). The effectiveness of community based rehabilitation for stroke patients who remain at home: a pilot randomised trial. *Clinical Rehabilitation* **14**, 563–9.

Young, J. and Forster, A. (1991). The Bradford community stroke trial: eight week results. *Clinical Rehabilitation* **5**, 283–92.

Young, J. and Forster, A. (1992). The Bradford community stroke trial: results at six months. *British Medical Journal* **304**, 1085–9.

Young, J. and Forster, A. (1993). Day hospital and home physiotherapy for stroke patients: a comparative cost-effectiveness study. *Journal of the Royal College of Physicians* **27**, 252–8.

8

Lessons from the South

Introduction

Community rehabilitation in the developed world is in its infancy. However, the less developed world (the South in modern terminology) has been using community-based rehabilitation services for at least 20 years. The purpose of this chapter is to describe community rehabilitation practice in the South and to explore whether any lessons can be learnt from that accumulated experience that can be put into place and developed in the North.

Epidemiology

Rehabilitation services are virtually nonexistent in many parts of the South despite huge, and increasing, numbers of disabled people. Estimates of disability amongst the global population have varied widely according to methods of survey and definitions of disability. However, the generally accepted figure (see Chapter 2) is around 10–14% of the total population. Many of these people have relatively mild disabilities and resources worldwide have tended to concentrate on those with more severe disabilities. The OPCS survey in the UK estimated that about 2–3% of the total population had a disability sufficiently severe to warrant the help from another individual at least once in every 24 hours (Martin et al., 1988). A significant proportion of moderately and severely disabled people are elderly and as life expectancy is less in the South it could be expected that the prevalence of more severe disability is also less. However, this demographic statistic has to be balanced against the higher rates of disability resulting from perinatal problems and communicable diseases. These two factors seem to balance each other and the prevalence of moderate and severe disability in the South probably lies around 4–5%

(Helander, 1993). A large-scale survey in China, for example, found 4.9% of the surveyed population had a significant disability – accounting for 18% of the surveyed households. This, in China alone, meant there were nearly 52 million significantly disabled people in that country at the time of the survey in 1987 (Ming and Jixiang, 1993). Other surveys found higher values in particular populations. The Zimbabwe National Disability Survey found that 15% was a reasonably accurate figure in that country (Davies, 1981). A total population surveyed in one village in Nigeria found 25% of the children aged 5–14 years to have some form of disability (Okunade, 1981). However, even if we accept that the prevalence figures of moderate and severe disability are broadly similar in the South and the North, disability still has a greater impact in the South considering that it affects a younger population. Disabled people are more likely to be either children or have young families, with consequently greater impact on society and the economy as a whole.

Regrettably, the magnitude of disability in Southern communities is increasing. It is estimated that by the year 2025 the number of people aged over 65 years living in the South will increase by about 212% (Helander, 1993). As life expectancy increases the proportion of disabled people in the population will also increase, worsening the situation in the less developed regions. Most of the world's population lives in the South and thus those countries are home to the great majority of the disabled global community. In 1975 it was estimated that 75% of the disabled population in the world lived in the South and this proportion is expected to rise still further (Noble, 1981). In actual numbers there were around 290 million disabled people in 1992 and this figure is estimated to rise to 573 million people in the world by 2025 (United Nations Development Programme, 1993). The numbers in the developed world are estimated to rise from 90 million to 138 million whereas the numbers in the less developed regions are estimated to rise from 200 million to 435 million over this timescale. Many of the disabilities prevalent in the South are potentially preventable, being secondary to complications in the perinatal period, communicable disease and the effects of accidents and malnutrition (United Nations Statistical Office, 1990).

These problems are compounded further by the virtual absence of organized rehabilitation services in the South. The South has simply not seen the growth of institutionally based rehabilitation services to the extent that has been witnessed in the North over the last 10–20 years. If services had developed along Northern lines then although many disabled people would not have had access to institutionally based regional centres nevertheless interest may have grown and expertise developed amongst the medical, nursing and therapy professions. Such expertise might, albeit slowly, have spread to the rural and isolated populations where most disabled people still live. However, the absence even of institutional rehabilitation has meant that most Southern countries do not have anybody with any significant rehabilitation background or skills. Thus, this has resulted not only in an absence of services, particularly for the rural populations, but also the absence of any significant lobbying or political voice in government circles. In general, Southern countries have had no history of the development of disability groups with any political clout. Thus, with a few notable exceptions, there has not only been no disability services but no government policy that might have changed the situation. The end result is that the overwhelming majority of disabled people in the South have no access at all to any rehabilitation services. In a comprehensive survey, for example, of 50 000 individuals in Pakistan, Miles (1981) found that 98% of the disabled population had received no help whatsoever. Other surveys reached similar conclusions. The World Health Organization has estimated that rehabilitation services are reaching no more than 2% of the total disabled population in the less developed regions (WHO, 1981).

This is a dire situation and it is perhaps surprising that any lessons can be drawn from rehabilitation experiences in the South. However, despite these overwhelming problems, developments have happened and have been largely through the intervention of nongovernmental organizations (NGOs), often working with the support of Northern-based aid organizations. This charitable-based approach to rehabilitation in the South is regrettable but nevertheless the flexibility and innovation that such organizations can bring has provided some lessons upon which we can draw.

Community-based rehabilitation

Rehabilitation in the South has largely developed along the lines originally suggested in the mid 1970s by the World Health Organization – a concept known as community-based rehabilitation or CBR. This concept grew out of increasing dissatisfaction and concern not only with the very limited resourcing of rehabilitation in the South but also with the inappropriateness of institutionally based rehabilitation. In 1976 the World Health Assembly adopted a resolution on disability, prevention and rehabilitation and made a strong case for increasing resources for disability programmes. The CBR concept is based on the idea that family members are the best resource for assisting with the daily needs of people with disabilities. The concept of CBR has, rightly, been adjusted and developed in different countries and different cultures and there is no universally accepted definition. Indeed the concept has been rather devalued by overusage and has been applied to any rehabilitation carried out in a community setting, whether that be a medically orientated hospital outreach programme or an initiative from within a local community. Early CBR projects, whilst recognizing the importance of family involvement, still largely had an impairment bias and focused mainly on the transference of basic rehabilitation techniques to community level workers. Most of the programmes could be considered as an extension of the institutional-based rehabilitation system. An example was the Government of India's National Leprosy Eradication Programme where emphasis was placed on treatment and restoration of function in people disabled by leprosy. This was largely an expert-based and outreach programme. India in the 1970s and 80s was one of the few countries to have a government strategy for disabled people. The government initiated a multidisciplinary rural rehabilitation programme called the District Rehabilitation Centre Scheme but this still emphasized medical intervention and outreach from institutions. The value of such schemes should not be underestimated but nevertheless they did little to build up either local expertise or involvement of the community. They also failed to develop the potential for economic self-sufficiency amongst the disabled population. Physical assistance, largely through aids and orthoses, was seen as an end in itself (Thomas and Thomas, 1999). Many CBR programmes still focus on the individual and improvement of personal functional abilities and some examples are given in later sections. However, in the late 1980s and early 1990s there was an increasing conceptual shift. In 1994 a joint position paper of the ILO, UNESCO and WHO redefined CBR as

A strategy within community development for the rehabilitation, equalization of opportunities and social integration of all people with disabilities. CBR is implemented through the combined efforts of disabled people themselves, their families and communities and the appropriate health, education, vocational and social services. (ILO, UNESCO and WHO, 1994)

Thus, with a stronger emphasis on the community and external societal factors there has been some shift in the nature of CBR projects. Many such projects now focus more on the provision of education for disabled people as well as education about the nature of disability for the family and local community. Many projects also focus on the development of economic self-sufficiency, often through collective groups of disabled people. The emphasis is much more on the societal disabling factors rather than simply on the improvement of individual functioning. However, the concept of CBR is still widely interpreted and many diverse activities are still given this label. CBR includes activities as wide-ranging as home-based services provided by families to their disabled members, self-help projects managed by disabled people themselves, outreach projects run by rehabilitation institutions, projects of nongovernmental organizations run by paid workers, institutional programmes located in villages or occasional outpatient clinics based in the community. It is important to emphasize that there is no 'right' model for CBR. Indeed rehabilitation is in need of a diverse and wide-ranging number of approaches. Community involvement and education is important but at the same time the development of health professional expertise is also vital in the long term. Thus, community projects should be developed hand in hand with health professional education, teaching and service delivery which is likely, at least initially, to be institutionally based. There is also a need for goodwill from governments, preferably backed up by governmental resources and legislation. It is likely that significant steps can only be taken when governments begin to view disabled people as having the same basic human rights as the able-bodied community.

Thus, CBR in the South represents a rich diversity of different concepts, ideologies and practice but with the unifying, underlying theme of local community involvement in the process. The next section gives some examples of CBR projects and highlights this diversity.

Examples of CBR projects

There are significant difficulties in giving examples of CBR projects around the world. Very few of the many thousands of projects are actually described or evaluated in the available literature. There is a clear tendency for successful projects to be written about whereas there is virtually no literature at all on projects that have failed. However, the lessons from the failed projects are just as important as the lessons from successful projects. It is a pity that there are very few journals that are prepared to publish simple descriptions of projects rather than detailed research evaluations. The number of projects that have been formally and rigorously evaluated are very few indeed.

A number of attempts have been made to classify CBR projects in order to help with discussion and evaluation. Murthy and Gopalan (1992) describe models of CBR based on aims of the programme – whether they be primarily health, education or economic. Peat and Boyce (1993) have described CBR services by focusing on the structure of the programme – whether it be outreach from an institution, dependent on local networks or as a service that simply promotes or facilitates CBR without actually offering direct clinical input. Other descriptions are based on the nature of those working within the programme – whether they be professional, semi-professional, persons with disabilities or local volunteers (Periquet, 1989). Others have taken a geographical focus – whether the programme is a national or a regional government programme, one supported by a nongovernmental organization either nationally or internationally, or whether the local community develops the programme (Kisanji, 1995). McColl and Patterson (1997) found it useful to describe CBR programmes using a framework based on six dimensions: the aims, strategies and beneficiaries that define the programme and the human, structural and attitudinal resources that support it. They constructed three-dimensional models using these parameters, which helped to represent each programme graphically and thus aid comparison between the different models. Their model allowed a specific programme to be situated in a three-dimensional graphic on the basis of the proportion of the stated aims, strategies and beneficiaries which were individually orientated as opposed to being community orientated. Similarly they were able to construct a three-dimensional model of support for each programme according to whether each of three factors (human, attitudinal and structural) drew mainly on support from inside or outside the targeted community. This work is a useful way to clarify the relationships between the many different approaches to CBR described in the literature.

The problem with any classification is that the nature of the programme often changes over time. A number of programmes have started with professional involvement on an outreach basis from a local institution and have grown to be more community focused with locally trained community volunteers taking on most of the rehabilitation work. Others have developed into educationally based projects and others aim towards economic self-sustainability. Many projects, of course, have a number of different aims and purposes running concurrently. In many ways the diversity and flexibility of CBR is the strength of the concept, but it does make it difficult for the projects to be described and evaluated. However, a few examples have been published or are personally known to the author. In broad and rather general terms the projects can be divided into three main categories.

First, there are projects that have grown from an institutional focus and are largely hospital outreach programmes, generally staffed by professionals working within a community setting. The second broad group are projects that are more firmly based in the local community often using locally trained workers, paid or voluntary, from the local community. Some of these projects continue to have a rehabilitation focus but others have developed broader aims including general health issues, such as clean water and vaccination. Others have begun to focus more broadly on income generation and economic self-sufficiency for disabled people. The third broad category are those projects that are not particularly involved in the actual delivery of health and rehabilitation services but are more focused on broader educational issues. These would include projects that concentrate on raising disability awareness both in the local community and for local leaders, such as teachers and primary healthcare staff.

Outreach CBR projects

It is doubtful whether institutional outreach projects can be compatible with CBR philosophy. Many have grown out of a realization that large numbers of disabled people are simply not able to access rehabilitation institutions, which are often based in centres of urban population. Such centres would normally exclude disabled people living in rural areas because of the cost and impracticability of travelling great distances. Thus, outpatient clinics are established in a local community setting and are staffed by professionals from the central institution. The concept of 'Camps', still prevalent in India, is a well-known example of such a scheme. Staff from a local rehabilitation centre or hospital will visit villages on a regular and preplanned basis to provide a range of outpatient-style health services. Obviously the focus can vary according to the specialism of those involved. Whilst one would not deny the practical importance of making health and rehabilitation services more available to local communities such projects do little to assist with the integration of disabled people into their local society nor would they have any particular impact on raising disability awareness or promoting economic self-sufficiency. However, many good-quality CBR projects have developed from such beginnings. In Bosnia Herzegovina, for example, the International Centre for the Advancement of Community Based Rehabilitation (ICACBR) has been at the forefront of development of outreach centres in postwar Bosnia. Very few health professional staff were left working in Bosnia in the postwar period and the new government felt that such expertise should be distributed as widely as possible. Thus, rehabilitation professional staff were available in 'ambulantas' which were local community clinics that provided a focus of service provision. This certainly represented a change in fundamental philosophy in ex-Yugoslavia as previously people with disabilities were treated in very large institutions, nearly always spending prolonged periods of time away from home and family. At the same time training programmes were initiated to increase the knowledge base and experience of local people, mainly from a professional health background, to work in such community clinics. However, it is important to note that a shift is occurring within these clinics. The shift is towards community participation, disability prevention and health education. Similar models are becoming prevalent in central and Eastern Europe. Marynika and colleagues (1991) describe the reorganization and restructuring of a typical village hospital in a rural part of the Ukraine. The Ukraine, in common with much of Eastern and central Europe, had previously provided rehabilitation in large centrally located tertiary centres. Local staff who were already based at the village hospital were given four months of additional rehabilitation training both at the regional centre and by staff from the regional centre providing on-site training. Some additional staff were hired including an instructor in exercise therapy and four rehabilitation nurses. Local people, through the local collective arrangements, funded changes to the physical structure of the hospital. In the year after the initiation the staff saw over 1000 disabled people, both on an outpatient basis and for brief periods of inpatient rehabilitation. The great majority of these people would never have received any rehabilitation services under the old system. The paper does not evaluate the quality of this service provision but nevertheless provides an interesting model for widening the population base for rehabilitation services in rural and relatively inaccessible communities.

Local CBR projects

Many projects have been started in the local community without links to regional and institutional bases. Probably the majority of CBR projects have started in this way through the initiatives of local NGOs with the support of foreign-based charitable organizations. Some have retained a purely rehabilitation focus whilst others have concentrated more on broader elements of primary healthcare and others have gone still wider into an educational and economic arena.

One of the few projects that has been written up in the world literature was described by Lagerkvist in 1992. The CBR programme had been running in the Philippines since about 1981. This was managed and supervised from a rehabilitation centre and was based on local supervisors acting as community workers. These had been recruited from the local villages and worked for 1–2 days a week with up to eight disabled people. The supervisors had had a short training for a few weeks based on the WHO training manual in CBR. The supervisors first identified the disabled people in house-to-house surveys and then started simple rehabilitation, working closely with the family. Referrals for further assessment and treatment were made to the local rehabilitation centre where professional rehabilitation staff were based. Over the first 6 years or so of the project a total of nearly 600 disabled people were under active rehabilitation in 53 villages with just over 100 local supervisors. This is one of the few projects which has had outcomes recorded. About a quarter of disabled children started school as a direct result of this intervention. The majority of disabled people had improved their level of physical functioning and improved integration into the local community.

Similar, and perhaps even better, results were obtained in another project in Zimbabwe described in the same paper. In Zimbabwe, the Zimbabwe Red Cross ran the CBR programme. This was a slightly different model, with two rehabilitation assistants with 1–2 years of medical education being responsible for assessment of the disabled people and drawing up a rehabilitation plan for each client. They also trained the local coordinators and volunteers who actually worked with the client in the villages. Thus, this was a more professionally orientated project but nevertheless still heavily relied on local people and family members to actually carry out the rehabilitation programme. In this programme about two-thirds of disabled children started school as a result of the intervention and about 50% of disabled men started work having previously been unemployed.

The Rural Aid project in Southern India is a further example. This project is run by a local NGO with the support of a British-based charitable organization, Action for Disability. The original focus for the project was a school for children with hearing impairment servicing an area of around 50 villages and a population of around 100 000 people. The area has virtually no healthcare access and certainly no rehabilitation services. It is a remote rural part of south India with very poor infrastructure. The school project leader identified the need for rehabilitation services, not only for children but also for adults. In this model the village 'dias' were recruited and paid on a part-time basis to act as rehabilitation assistants. The 'dias' are local women, usually one per village, who effectively act as midwives for the local community. They underwent training of a few weeks, supervised by multipurpose health workers who each covered around 10–15 villages. Training was largely in basic concepts of rehabilitation for people with physical disabilities but also encompassed similar basic concepts of primary healthcare such as clean water, vaccination and better quality antenatal and postnatal care. The multipurpose health workers provided rehabilitation for those with more complex disabilities and a few of those people were referred onwards to the local hospital and even to the regional rehabilitation centre based around 200 kilometres away in Vellore. Over a period of 3–4 years most of the villages developed disability self-help groups. These groups meet on a regular basis and each member contributes a small amount to a central mini-bank which is then used to buy aids and equipment for members of their own group and to pay for referral to the local hospital or rehabilitation centre. The groups are also slowly becoming more economically self-sufficient and have started a variety of projects including farming, sari weaving and basket work. The project still requires external support for both the deaf school and the orthotic workshop and for the salaries of the multipurpose health workers.

This slowly evolving diversification is quite a common theme among CBR projects. Similar experiences have been documented in the Solomon Islands (Hill et al., 1997), Ghana (Kassah, 1998) and the Philippines (Ortali, 2000).

Other CBR projects have started from a disability awareness raising and disability educational perspective (Miles, 1996). Such projects often involve disabled people right from the beginning in the creation of the disability group within the local community. The members of the group then decide on the priorities, which may be health- or rehabilitation-related or may focus more on educational needs and income-generating projects. An example is the SACRED project in Andhra Pradesh in rural southern India. This project was started by one individual who had been trained in CBR by Action Aid in India as well as a training course in London, England. The individual encouraged the formation of disability groups within the local area initially starting with just six groups in villages surrounding the town of Anantapur. The assistance of the British- based charity, Action for Disability, was enlisted and three more community rehabilitation workers were recruited and trained by the project coordinator. The project therefore was able to cover a broader geographical area and further disability self-help groups were established in more villages. Over a 3-year period a total of about 50 villages (population around 100 000) were covered. The groups were encouraged to form mini-banks and develop and implement ideas for income generation. Most groups now run their own small income-generating projects, including tailoring, poultry farming and fruit growing. Simple rehabilitation input is given by the community rehabilitation workers but with the support and input of the disability group and families. The mini-bank scheme pays for simple disability aids and for the occasional referral to the local health centre or hospital. The project now has a community centre that acts as an educational and training base and houses a simple orthotic workshop.

A similar programme, on a larger scale, has been initiated in Afghanistan. The United Nations Development Programme (UNDP) set up the Comprehensive Disabled Afghan's Programme in 1995. This large national programme now operates in 13 provinces employing some 400 paid staff and several hundred volunteers. It provides input to over 27 000 disabled people annually. The key agents in the field are mid-level rehabilitation workers, both male and female. They each cover a population of between 15–30 000. Their role is to activate local CBR committees and disabled people's organizations, recruit volunteers, identify disabled people through local surveys and arrange appropriate services for each disabled person. However, the project is broader than simple health and rehabilitation input. There is a focus on integrating disabled children into local schools and providing training and employment for disabled adults. Loans can be given to establish small businesses and to attend skills training courses. Referrals can be made if necessary to physiotherapy centres or the local orthopaedic workshops. The mid-level rehabilitation workers are given 5 months training in community development, psychology, child development, teaching and learning skills as well as basic rehabilitation principles and practice. These workers are supported by smaller groups of specialists including physiotherapists, orthopaedic technicians, employment specialists and educationalists. The mid-level rehabilitation workers themselves are supported by up to five volunteers each.

An important aspect of the programme is information, education and communication, which aims to raise disability issues within Afghanistan through newsletters, radio broadcasts, posters, videos, leaflets and discussion groups.

CBR educational programmes

Some programmes are set up entirely as educational and disability awareness projects, although most of the CBR projects will have an educative element. A project in Palestine (Union of Palestinian Medical Relief Committees; described in Peat, 1997) was established with a primary educational focus. The aim was to raise general disability consciousness and build awareness for both people with disabilities and their communities at large. The organization facilitates education, employment and vocational training for people with disabilities. It provides teaching and education input for school teachers as well as providing an educational forum in the communities themselves. This organization has now developed to provide training for community rehabilitation workers and the focus has shifted somewhat to assist people with disabilities to live independently by skills training courses in local community resource centres. There has been little direct personal rehabilitation support. A similar organization in Kenya (African Medical and Research Foundation; described in Peat, 1997) has remained purely educational. The objective of this organization is to increase awareness of the need for and importance of early detection, intervention and prevention of disability in the community. It also trains teachers and community health workers in simple rehabilitation skills, knowledge and attitude as well as organizing and facilitating vocational training courses.

Thus, we can see that there is a wide range of CBR projects involving different levels of rehabilitation, health education, vocational and independence training. The projects are delivered through a variety of individuals from fully trained professional doctors, nurses and therapists to less qualified generic health workers and briefly trained local village and community workers. However, the unifying theme of the projects is the direct involvement of disabled people in the planning and implementation of the programme as well as involvement of the family and local community in the delivery of the service. There is also a common theme that most projects, from whatever starting point, have moved towards broadbased programmes with a realization that individual rehabilitation is of limited value without local social support, education and economic self-sufficiency.

Lessons to be learnt

CBR projects in the South are geared to the local, cultural, political, economic and health situation. Most of these factors are very significantly different in the more developed nations. Thus, are there any lessons that can be learnt from CBR work that may be applicable to community rehabilitation development in the North? Undoubtedly general lessons can be learnt from these various experiences that can be directly applicable when planning community rehabilitation in better resourced countries. What are these lessons?

Participation by disabled people

The very clear lesson from the majority of CBR projects is that for the project to have acceptance by and meaning for the disabled population there must be the participation of people with disabilities at all stages. This should mean that local disabled people have a clear and direct stake, even at the very early planning stages, regarding the sort of service that should be established in their own locality. If disabled groups do not exist then health planners and health professionals should clearly encourage such groups to come together. This is relatively straightforward if disease-specific teams are being established. If, for example, a community multiple sclerosis team is being planned then it is often fairly straightforward for the local branch of the MS Society to be consulted and be actively involved in the design and planning of the service. However, problems can well arise if a rehabilitation team is being established with a more broadbased disability focus covering a variety of diagnoses. In many places there are simply no disability groups that can be consulted. The lessons from the South certainly indicate that if this is the case then every attempt should be made to establish such a group or at least to assemble a number of interested disabled people whether or not they would be personally affected by the service. Preferably the disabled group should not only be part of the planning process but be an active partner in the continued monitoring of the project on a management or steering group.

Community participation

Many societies in the South are firmly based around the family with mutual support between extended family members. This is less so in many Northern societies where family mobility and geographical spread are more common and families are less in touch and less likely to support disabled members. However, it is still possible and desirable for community rehabilitation programmes to involve the broader community at large. In practical terms this may mean involving local community leaders in the planning and implementation of a project. It may mean that the physical base for the rehabilitation service should be in a local community centre or it may mean that disability awareness and specific information programmes are advertised and conducted in accessible local facilities. Educational programmes could be put on in local schools and local employers could be involved in the process of encouraging disabled people into work. The community can provide a resource of volunteers and sometimes financial support. Any attempt to involve the able-bodied community should be encouraged with the long-term aim of improved social integration of people with disabilities.

Primary care focus

Another lesson to be learnt is that it is unrealistic to provide rehabilitation in a local community without adequate primary care and a public health programme. Disabled people, as well as able-bodied community members, need primary healthcare as well as health education about such basic considerations as clean water and a vaccination programme. Ideally the rehabilitation worker should be part of a community-based primary-care team. However, where no primary health service exists then it is important for the rehabilitation worker to be trained in the basic principles of primary healthcare. Simple measures to promote improved childbirth, sensible use of antibiotics, clean water and vaccination will not only help the entire local community but will contribute in the longer term to the reduction of disability. In the North we are seeing the further development of primary care (Edmonds and Peat, 1997). In the UK the GP is becoming the focus for the NHS. Community rehabilitation should be an integral part of this drive for improved local primary healthcare services.

Flexibility

The great majority of CBR projects in the South have changed, often significantly, over time as needs and priorities are identified and the situations change. The role and remit of the local community team need to remain flexible and the service will often need adjusting as experience develops. Rigidity of thought and management style are to be actively discouraged.

Avoidance of professional boundaries

The wholly different economic situation in the South dictates that fully trained health professionals cannot support the great majority of CBR programmes. Whilst the situation is different in the North it remains unlikely that each locality can have a full multidisciplinary team serving the full needs of disabled people and staffed only by qualified health professionals. There are simply not enough such people to go around. Many CBR projects in the South have shown the value of broader-based generic training. There is surprising consistency amongst the reports published that demonstrate that generic workers without reference to specialist professionals can serve about 80% of rehabilitation needs. There are many models that can be used in the North. Some countries have seen the advent, albeit on a small scale, of therapy assistants who work on the ground under the occasional supervision of a qualified therapist. Such individuals largely exist within the realms of physiotherapy and occupational therapy. In the UK there has been the growth of the nurse practitioner who is further trained in a specialist area, such as multiple sclerosis, epilepsy or diabetes, and who takes on the role of generic rehabilitation worker – dealing with most difficulties alone but with the ability to refer to relevant specialists as required. Some countries make use of volunteers. There is so far no real concept anywhere in the world

of the generic rehabilitation worker who is a 'specialist' in their own right
with their own recognized national training programme. Perhaps such individuals would provide a more holistic approach to disability dealing with
the whole persons' needs rather than compartmentalizing disability according to professional divisions. CBR training programmes in the South have
shown that a basic, practical and safe training can be delivered in about
3 months, which would be sufficient to provide a reasonable rehabilitation
input to most disabled people, albeit under the guidance of more fully trained
specialists.

Cultural diversity

Most developed countries, particularly in urban areas, now have a diverse
multicultural mix. Interpretation of the attitude to disability varies widely
between cultures and religions and any community rehabilitation project
must take into account the cultural and religious background of the local
community. As a minimum this means providing good quality information
in the relevant language but should more positively mean that those disabled
people from different ethnic backgrounds or representatives from different
ethnic communities should also be involved in the planning and supervision
of the service.

Educational and economic focus

Many community rehabilitation teams will be funded and supported by the
government department of health and thus most will clearly need to have a
health and rehabilitation focus. However, the lessons from the South show
that whilst individual rehabilitation is important it is equally important to
provide broader education, educational opportunities and opportunities for
independent living and economic self-sufficiency. In practical terms this
may mean that the local team could take a role in lobbying for better physical
access in the vicinity or better integration between health and social services
or for greater numbers of disabled children to be properly integrated into
local mainstream schools. Adults could be encouraged to take part in adult
learning opportunities and the local educationalists equally encouraged to
advertise and make accessible such courses to the disabled community. Local
employers could be targeted to take on more disabled employees and the local
disability group could certainly take a lead in more active political lobbying

to increase disability awareness and put more resources towards relevant disability services.

Information is the key to independence and the community rehabilitation team should provide a whole range of relevant and understandable literature not only about various disease states but also about symptom management, as well as information on local resources and facilities.

Some pitfalls of Southern CBR projects

There are also some pitfalls that can be avoided from the Southern experience. There is a real risk of a patchy community rehabilitation service unless there is some coordination of planning. As an example in Newcastle upon Tyne there is an excellent community multiple sclerosis team as well as community rehabilitation teams servicing the elderly population. However, younger people with disabilities other than multiple sclerosis have no access to any specific community rehabilitation. In a neighbouring locality there is a community head-injury team but no other specific disorder is served by any community rehabilitation other than the rather patchy availability of community physiotherapy and occupational therapy. Some would argue that too much community emphasis may dilute specialist expertise and devalue the role of institutional regional centres. It should be emphasized that many CBR projects in the South still need the active involvement and support of specialized professionals and often people will need referral to specialist centres. Both such services are needed – one is not a substitute for the other.

The primary pitfall that should be avoided in the North is a lack of research and dissemination of such research. The vast majority of CBR projects in the South have never been evaluated and even the few that have are available only in internal reports for various funding bodies. The research literature in this field available to the general public is minimal. Any new community rehabilitation project should be encouraged to undergo an audit and preferably for such audit, whether good or bad, to be published and made widely available so that lessons can be learnt and progress made.

Conclusion

Overall, community-based rehabilitation has made significant strides in the South over the last 20 years or so. There are many lessons that can be learnt and pitfalls avoided by studying those projects. The key lesson is that the involvement of disabled people and the local community in project planning and implementation is a requirement for the success of the project.

REFERENCES

Davies, M.P. (1981). Zimbabwe National Disability Survey. *African's Rehabilitation Journal* **1**, 1.

Edmonds, L.J. and Peat, M. (1997). Community based rehabilitation (CBR) and health reform: a timely strategy. *Canadian Journal of Rehabilitation* **10**, 273–83.

Helander, E. (1993). *Prejudice and Dignity: An Introduction to Community Based Rehabilitation.* New York: United Nations Development Programme.

Hill, L., McAuley, C., Sarchuk, C. and Shalom, L. (1997). Community based rehabilitation in Solomon Islands: lessons learned by Canadian rehabilitation professionals. *Canadian Journal of Rehabilitation* **10**, 285–95.

ILO, UNESCO and WHO (1994). *Community Based Rehabilitation for and with People with Disabilities.* Joint Position Paper. New York: United Nations.

Kassah, A.K. (1998). Community based rehabilitation and stigma management by physically disabled people in Ghana. *Disability and Rehabilitation* **20**, 66–73.

Kisanji, J. (1995). Understanding community based rehabilitation models. *CBR News* **19**, 4.

Lagerkvist, B. (1992). Community based rehabilitation – outcome for the disabled in the Philippines and Zimbabwe. *Disability and Rehabilitation* **14**, 44–50.

Martin, J., Meltzer, H. and Elliot, D. (1988). *The Prevalence of Disability among Young Adults.* OPCS Report 1. London: HMSO.

Marynika, O., Ovcharenko, A., Pelekh, L. and Palamarchuk, L. (1991). Rehabilitation in a rural community in Ukraine – a pilot project. *International Disability Studies* **13**, 20–2.

McColl, M.A. and Patterson, J. (1997). A descriptive framework for community based rehabilitation. *Canadian Journal of Rehabilitation* **10**, 297–306.

Miles, M. (1981). *Mis-planning for Disabilities in Asia.* Peshawar, Pakistan: Private publication.

Miles, S. (1996). Engaging with the disability rights movement: the experience of community based rehabilitation in Southern Africa. *Disability and Society* **11**, 501–17.

Ming, G. and Jixiang, M. (1993). Demography of people with disabilities in China. *International Journal of Rehabilitation Research* **16**, 299–301.

Murthy, S.P. and Gopalan, L. (1992). *Workbook on Community Based Rehabilitation Services.* Bangalore: Action Aid.

Noble, J.H. (1981). Social inequity and the prevalence for disability, projections for the year 2000. *Assignment Children* **53/54**, 23–32.

Okunade, J. (1981). Youruba attitudes to the handicapped. *Child Care Health and Development* **7**, 187–94.

Ortali, F. (2000). Analysis of multi-sectoral collaboration in community based rehabilitation. *Asia Pacific Disability Rehabilitation Journal* **11**, 86–94.

Peat, M. (1997). *Community Based Rehabilitation.* London: WB Saunders.

Peat, M. and Boyce, W. (1993). Canadian community rehabilitation services. Challenges for the future. *Canadian Journal of Rehabilitation* **6**, 281–9.

Periquet, A.O. (1989). Community based rehabilitation in the Philippines. *International Disability Studies* **11**, 95–6.

Thomas, M. and Thomas, M.J. (1999). A discussion on the shifts and changes in community based rehabilitation in the last decade. *Neural Rehabilitation and Neural Repair* **13**, 185–9.

United Nations Development Programme (1993). *Disabled People's Participation in Sustainable Human Development.* New York: Division for Global and Inter-Regional Programmes, UNDP.

United Nations Statistical Office (1990). *Disabilities, Statistics, Database and Compendium.* New York: UNSO.

World Health Organisation (1981). *Global Strategy of Health for All by the Year 2000.* (Health for All Series 3). Geneva: WHO.

9

Other aspects of community neurological rehabilitation

Overview

If someone has been diagnosed with multiple sclerosis, sustained a stroke or is living with cerebral palsy, medical and therapeutic intervention is likely to form a substantial part of his or her life. The extent to which it does is dependent on the individual. At the acute end of the spectrum, health-related intervention is likely to be a priority as individuals may be in critical conditions. In the community, individuals may still have impairment-related needs, but they are likely to extend beyond the medical domain.

Neurological impairments not only affect an individual's physical and emotional health, but they can impact on many other areas of life. This includes employment, housing, education, transport and sport and leisure activities. Informal support networks, such as family and friends, may also play a significant part in the lives of disabled people. While rehabilitative practice focuses on health-related needs, many governmental agencies in the North are obliged to meet these additional social needs, including the needs of carers. In the past these needs have often been met in isolation in a number of different ways owing to the organizational structure of the different agencies involved and the source of funding. This has resulted in long delays, bad coordination, lack of communication, gaps and overlap in services, inefficient use of limited resources, inappropriate services, lack of flexibility and ultimately confusion for the client (Beardshaw, 1988).

The growing emphasis placed on more abstract concepts such as 'quality of life' which demand a more holistic approach to providing rehabilitation is an acknowledgement that disabled people do have more than just health-related needs, and that they need to be addressed together. This entails a more client-centred approach. Knowledge of a client's broader range of needs may serve to inform the rehabilitative process and have implications for its more effective delivery. Thus the aim of this chapter is to put health-related factors into perspective by outlining the other factors that also hold high priorities for disabled people. However, it should be noted that the following serves purely as an outline which is unlikely to touch upon all the intricate issues that are involved, especially those of cultural variations.

Employment

A man willing to work, and unable to find work, is perhaps the saddest sight that fortune's inequality exhibits under the sun. Thomas Carlisle (1795–1881)

Unemployment is a cause of low self-esteem for many people. This is especially true for disabled people, who often may have the appropriate skills but are unable to find work due to a range of attitudinal and physical barriers. Our society is such that work or training occupies much of our time, and through this we not only afford our living costs but also construct our sense of identity. 'At work, people are a part of a complex set of complementary relationships which convey identity and status. All this is lost in unemployment' (Argyle, 1967).

Epidemiology

In the UK, disabled people are over six times as likely as nondisabled people to be out of work and claiming benefits. Furthermore, over 2.6 million disabled people were noted to be out of work and on benefits, with over a million of them wanting to work. In America, the unemployment rate for people with disabilities is 72%; of those, 67% want to work (Partners in Policy Making, 1993). A Dutch study noted that well over 20% of the working-age population in the Netherlands is partially or totally incapacitated for work due to illness, chronic disorders or other limitations (van Lierop and Nijhuis, 2000). In Sweden, of 195 people who were employed before a stroke or traumatic brain injury, only 25% returned to their previous jobs after 3 years and 20% of these had different work tasks (Soderback et al., 1991). The difficulty for workers who have been incapacitated for more than 2 years to find re-employment is widely recognized. These statistics, among many others, clearly support the demand for more work-related measures to improve the opportunities for disabled people to find employment. Some of these measures have been documented and will be described below.

Employment programmes

These programmes differ in that some aim to train individuals prior to placement (vocational training), whereas others work towards an immediate placement followed by training (employer-based rehabilitation). Another system, which has been referred to as 'supported' employment, attempts to enable people to work through the further employment of personal assistants. Research about disability and employment is a neglected area (Floyd, 1991), but the following descriptions attempt to bring together some of the literature to illustrate the types of programmes available.

Vocational training programmes (train, then place)

A centre running a holistic psychosocial rehabilitation programme for individuals with postacute traumatic brain injury in Denmark emphasized return to employment or education as a major target for the programme (Christensen, 1992). The programme had two phases; the first required its clients to come to the centre for 6 hours a day, 4 days a week, for a period of about 4 months. A structured timetable was set up for each individual dependent on specific needs and interests, but involved a range of individual and group work. There was also close contact with family members, ensuring that they also received the chance to voice their concerns and gain the support they required. The second phase concerned the ongoing future of each client, specifically relating to the practical opportunities for employment or education. This was tied in with follow-up group sessions which provided a chance for individuals to exchange their experiences. Desirable outcomes were rated as those who at posttreatment or follow-up were engaged in education, a work trial or gainful employment. Of the first 46 clients that completed the programme there was a significant improvement between pre- and posttreatment; almost 20% of them returned to gainful employment at the pre-injury level. Thus the findings strongly suggested that participation in the treatment programme enhanced the prospect of a return to employment or an education programme and of sustaining that return (Christensen, 1992).

This programme shares characteristics with that of a vocational training organization, Rehab UK, that currently has five centres in the UK. They provide adults with brain-injuries specialist rehabilitation services in order to gain, regain and sustain employment. The average length of each programme is 38 weeks and this is divided into three main phases: (1) assessment, induction, exploration and core skills; (2) centre-based training and development; and (3) work placement and job coaching. In one of its sites, 76.5% of clients during 1 year had been successfully integrated into employment, voluntary work or further education (i.e. attained a 'hard' outcome). Thus, far from being a cost to the exchequer these individuals become contributors, both in productivity and in payment of taxes. An evaluation of the newest branch of Rehab UK has not produced such positive outcomes (28% attained a 'hard' outcome, as defined above), which may be due to it being a relatively new enterprise in the area, with the remaining clients still being on placements or training. The main reason for work-placement breakdown was the slow acquisition of job skills. Other reasons may be associated with faults in the referral process and misperceptions about the aim of the centre.

Success of vocational programmes is typically based upon the number of people who, after training, join the competitive labour market. The first study in the Netherlands to investigate the long-term effectiveness of vocational rehabilitation programmes did so in three different centres (van Lierop and Nijhuis, 2000). All of the centres provided certified occupational training, personal skills training and counselling to potentially active workers who had lost contact with the labour market. After 5 years it was found that 80% of the trainees were working in the competitive labour market, with a significant improvement in their personal skills. Meanwhile in Italy 44 unemployed people with brain injuries undertook a course of vocational training in the use of computers, computerized neuropsychological rehabilitation and physical stamina training over a period of 6 months. Following training they were given placements, and 6 months later about half of them were employed either as professionals, civil servants or in private firms (Perino et al., 2000). Thus economic advantage is experienced not only by individuals themselves, but also for society as a whole.

Employer-based rehabilitation (place, then train)

The vocational programmes described above have been shown to produce some positive outcomes, in terms of getting people back into meaningful occupations. However, within the current dynamics of the labour market and the inevitable drive towards cost-effectiveness, even this method can prove to be time consuming and costly. Employer-based rehabilitation not only aims to get clients back to work in the shortest time possible, but is also sensitive to the nature of the labour market. The principle is to incorporate rehabilitation plans within a work setting. This 'in-context' assessment has been tested and proven to be effective (Lougheed, 1998). The benefits of this type of assessment are many. First, by placing clients directly into the working environment they experience higher levels of self-esteem, serving to facilitate and strengthen the rehabilitative process. Second, this testing has excellent face validity, in that it measures what it is designed to measure. Third, the predictive value of the assessment is high because the work skills and work behaviours that are likely to be required have been assessed directly.

Another factor that is crucial to employer-based rehabilitation is motivation. If a client is not motivated to work then it will be very difficult to get any work done effectively. Motivation is inextricably linked with beliefs of self-efficacy; as research indicates, activities will only be followed through if we believe that we are capable of doing them (Betz and Hackett, 1981). Hence a primary goal is to enhance individual self-efficacy. This is achieved in such assessments by helping each client to rate their own capacity for each identified work demand. Following the completion of an employer-based assessment, clients' self-efficacy beliefs are defined and they have greater self-awareness together with a list of transferable skills (Lougheed, 1998).

In Sweden there are several occupational work-training programmes but little evaluation has been done on them (Soderback et al., 1993). The role of the occupational therapist is to work within a team to assess individual needs, resources, problems and barriers in relation to employment. Soderback described an innovative programme that was divided into five different phases. This included assessment, job analyses, work training and continuous evaluation. The programmes were adapted to the individual, and started from the point at which the individual arrived at the neurosurgical ward to the time when his/her maximal ability had been reached. This procedure appeared to be of value to the participants.

Supported employment

Supported employment is another system by which severely disabled people are enabled to work. Disabled individuals are allocated with a personal assistant who is employed to make working in an ordinary job environment possible. This programme is most commonly associated with learning-disabled people, but could easily be applied to those with neurological impairments. The interesting feature of this system is that it is not assumed that individuals will ever work entirely independently, and hence it might seem bizarre that two individuals are employed to carry out one task. However, due to budgetary arrangements, and the benefits of keeping people out of special institutions and occupied in more meaningful environments, this system is deemed to be ultimately cost-efficient (Devlieger, 1999).

It has been noted that the more supported employment programmes simulate real job environments, the more they will be experienced as such (Mank et al., 1997) and hence are more likely to have a positive outcome. Therefore any programme that reinforces the 'job coach' model may be in danger of obstructing the path towards a positive outcome. Trach and Shelden (1999) promote the use of a variety of 'natural supports' that aim to achieve successful employment, beyond merely job retention, to provide a basis from which supported employment can develop. Despite the extent of published work that documents the successes of supported employment, its impact on the unwaveringly high unemployment rate among disabled people remains minimal (Wehman and Revell, 1998).

Sheltered employment

Sheltered employment does not constitute successful reintegration into the competitive labour market. Individuals enrolled in such programmes are occupied within a controlled environment, usually carrying out simple and repetitive tasks. This attempts to simulate the working environment under the management of an independent body, in isolation from the labour force. In the North this practice is largely outdated now, losing popularity for ethical reasons.

Summary

The programmes described so far are in their infancy, and the literature tends to be descriptive rather than rigorously evaluative. Due to ethical considerations it is not possible to have a control group, and thus more creative and variable methodological techniques are generally required. While each programme may have its advantages, without further evaluation it is not possible to identify these in more detail. As is often the case, reports of failed or unsuccessful programmes are unlikely to be documented which would otherwise inform the developmental process.

There are many other issues that might also prescribe the success of a programme. Even though working with a previous employer is more likely to be successful than in a new environment (Johnson, 1987), people from professional backgrounds are less likely to succeed in any employment programme due to having reduced levels of responsibility (Wehman and Kreutzer, 1994: cited in Ponsford et al., 1996). Timing of employment is crucial and largely dependent on the individual, but it is nevertheless important to start planning it at an early stage (Ponsford et al., 1996). Programmes not only need to overcome barriers to finding jobs, but also to maintain people in jobs once found. Individuals with traumatic brain injury frequently have less difficulty in finding employment than in maintaining it (Kreutzer and Morton, 1988: cited in Ponsford et al., 1996). This can be for reasons involving interpersonal relationships, conflicts with fellow workers, lack of interest, poor attendance, low motivation or transportation problems.

In the quest to find more effective procedures what can be deduced is that every programme demands individual tailoring. Thus it might be unrealistic to expect there to be one ultimate programme guaranteed to suit all. Further research is required to investigate which elements of programmes are most associated with successful outcomes, and to examine their interactions between different personality characteristics (van Lierop and Nijhuis, 2000). However, employment opportunities remain limited as long as the medical model dominates both the literature and practice (Duckett, 2000). In this way it is nearly always the individual who is targeted for change, as illustrated by the studies above that train individuals to improve their social skills, interview skills, motivation or communication. Adopting research methods that also take into consideration the impact of the environment may lead to less discriminatory practice and hence further opportunities for disabled people. This has been an issue high on the agenda for those working within the social model of disability, that targets society as being the barrier to equal opportunities. The studies below illustrate these advances.

Barriers to employment

An ongoing research project conducted in London is investigating the barriers to and factors facilitating employment after stroke. It is a collaborative project between the research team and members of Different Strokes, an organization of younger stroke survivors. The project is divided into four parts, using both qualitative and quantitative methods, and it is committed to maximizing the active participation of stroke survivors themselves. Stage one involved focus groups with stroke survivors, and served to inform the development of a questionnaire (stage two) to be sent to 3000 stroke survivors. In-depth interviews are being planned with a subset of these participants to explore personal experience and verify the earlier findings. The final stage is to incorporate the views of employers themselves, highlighting the issues that have been raised across the lifetime of the project.

Breakthrough UK, an organization set up to provide training and employment and business opportunities to disabled people, have recently carried out a similar study (Branfield and Maynard Campbell, 2000). They employ a social model approach in their practice and research, asserting that if the barriers to employment and training are created by society then they can also be removed by society. These barriers fall loosely into three categories: environmental and physical, attitudinal and organizational or institutional. The findings revealed that regardless of a disabled person's ability, experience or background, a range of discriminatory practices are encountered when they attempt to find work or training. These include poor transport, inaccessible buildings, poor access to information, negative attitudes, inflexible practices, delays for equipment and limited opportunities for disability equality training. One man stated 'I have always had difficulty getting a job. It's like they see a leper coming', while a comment by another person illustrates that even once you get a job there is no guarantee of keeping it: 'I was told that I was not being dismissed. I was told that it wasn't working out but I wasn't given a reason and it was a complete shock.' Research such as this exposes the real difficulties that disabled people face every day. Since the Disability Discrimination Act (1995) in the UK and the Americans with Disabilities Act (1990) in the USA were put in place there has been little evidence of better employment prospects (Duckett, 2000). Disabled people are a heterogeneous group with many different kinds of impairments. People with neurological impairments are discriminated against particularly harshly (Gouvier and Steiner, 1991).

More acknowledgement of the range of needs is required to make useful and permanent changes.

Future prospects

While the studies above have tended to portray employment-related programmes in a positive light, the lack of literature means that our understanding of their success is limited. Given that disabled people are often discriminated against in terms of gaining meaningful employment, it paves the way for examining this situation in much greater depth. It is evident, for example, that there is a need for more competitive and noncompetitive work options, including the possibility of volunteer work (Jackson, 1994). Governments will soon be obliged (if they are not already) to offer many more opportunities on the grounds of equal human rights (Human Rights Act, 1998). This is despite the fact that it is actually in their favour to make changes to this effect, considering the higher tax returns and lower outgoings (in relation to benefits). As it stands at present, legislation will determine whether disabled people have the incentive to work. There may be considerable international variation, due to the political and economical climates, but it is evident that both employment and disability are issues worldwide and further collaboration and research in this area will no doubt be of value.

Housing

The importance of having somewhere to live, and ultimately somewhere we can call home, is an issue for us all. Most housing is built with the dimensions of the average human being in mind and this does not usually cater for those in wheelchairs and other mobility impairments. While this was not so much an issue in the past, when disabled people were mostly segregated into specially adapted accommodation or institutions, the move towards rehabilitation in the community has meant an increase in demand for adequate housing and individual adaptations. Hence, for disabled people to achieve their full potential in the community, housing needs to be given a higher priority (Dunn, 1990). This may be in the form of a private household, some form of supported living scheme such as supervised housing, shared services, foster care (Jackson, 1994) or a transitional living programme.

The steady transition of disabled people from institutions to the community has been of interest to governmental agencies on a number of levels.

Research into people with learning impairments has found that there may be savings to be made in community-based programmes as opposed to state institutions (Knobbe et al., 1995). Furthermore, Heller et al. (1999) found that of those adults with cerebral palsy who made the transition from nursing homes to community-based settings, their health status, mobility limitations and community inclusion improved, while there was no significant change for nonmovers.

Further research has shown that an accessible housing environment was not only supportive for health reasons, but also beneficial to gaining independence in daily life (Dunn, 1990; Iwarsson and Isacsson, 1997; Iwarsson, 1999). The development of an objective tool for assessing accessibility, the 'Housing Enabler' (Iwarsson and Isacsson, 1996), was among the first tools available within a community environment. Since then a self-administered instrument to be used in conjunction with the Housing Enabler has been developed to gain insight into the client's own perception of accessibility (Fange and Iwarsson, 1999). Being able to assess accessibility in this way may have implications for other aspects of life, such as public transport, research and education, and is an important advance in the realization that rehabilitation not only involves changing the individual but changing his/her environment.

In summary, better housing options for disabled people are likely to benefit their health and general lifestyle. This is not only positive for disabled people themselves, but also for the governments for whom it is also cost-effective. With this in mind, housing policies need to be enforced and adapted so as to respond to the needs of disabled people (Dunn, 1990).

Sport and leisure

Too great an emphasis on the goals of independence, mobility and self-care within disciplines such as physiotherapy and occupational therapy can lead to the exclusion of other related needs. Sport and leisure pursuits are integral to many people's lives and yet even when individuals have made good physical recoveries they show a particular decrease in time spent in such activities (Parker et al., 1997). In his criticism of rehabilitation, where people tend not to be treated as individuals with thoughts and feelings, and where services are slow to materialize at critical times, Bathurst (1999) has emphasized the importance of providing positive messages to people about the future. He refers to a 'leisure education model' which would seek to provide support in setting goals and promoting self-determination, taking the focus away from the therapy aspect. He recognizes that people need respite from therapy; to have at least some part of their life that is not pathologized. A form of 'specialized' occupational therapy, with leisure enhancement as its primary goal, may be one way in which to boost leisure activity and the pursuit of enjoyment, and consequently psychological well-being (Drummond and Walker, 1996). This reflects the finding that leisure satisfaction has been found to contribute most to satisfaction in community life (Allen and Beattie, 1984). Despite the recent development of objective measuring instruments, such as the Nottingham Leisure Questionnaire (Drummond and Walker, 1994), more research would be needed to confirm this correlation. The most recent study of its kind failed to support the routine use of leisure therapy in the community for its beneficial effects on mood and leisure participation (Parker et al., 2001).

There are many obstacles that hinder the widescale pursuit of enjoyment-seeking activities. In elderly people especially, lack of personal transport, inadequate finance, physical impairment and fear all contribute to the noticeable decline in such activities (Parker et al., 1997). However, if these and other barriers such as low self-esteem, reluctance of carers and societal attitudes can be overcome then the benefits of sport and leisure can be appreciated by all.

Sport instils self-discipline, a competitive spirit and comradeship, along with opportunities to establish social contacts (Chawla, 1994). The growing interest in competitive sports at an Olympic level for disabled people is an indication of its importance. As with able-bodied events guidelines are drawn up and this enables participants with a wide range of impairments to compete on equal terms. As long as disabled people have access to medical advice and regular reviews then there is every reason for promoting these activities. In the context of rehabilitation, there is a need to reconfigure the boundaries in which therapies on offer are viewed: leisure being a simple extension of occupational therapy, and sport an extension of physiotherapy.

Transport and driving

In modern society, being able to drive a car can be the key to independence (Barnes and Hoyle, 1995). For disabled people it may be essential where access to public transport is often difficult. However, access to driving assessments, advice on ability to drive and car adaptation are not easy to arrange. In a study to investigate the demand for such a service, Barnes and Hoyle (1995) found that at least 20% of the disabled population proposed that driving assessment and advice should be an integral part of the rehabilitative process. In the neurologically disabled population poor judgement, impulsivity and visuospatial impairments are common problems that traditional assessments are ill-equipped to measure (van Zomeren et al., 1987). Before driving can become more accessible to disabled people, there is a need for standardized, reliable and specific scoring criteria to ascertain any deficiencies in driving skills that may be amenable to training (Fox et al., 1998).

There are now numerous adaptations to enable even the most severely disabled person to drive a motor vehicle. Adaptations range from the simple and cheap to the complex and expensive. For many disabled people purchase of a car with a wide entry door and automatic transmission is sufficient to reduce the problems of getting in and out and car control. Individuals with impaired leg function can usually easily manage with automatic transmission and hand controls. Individuals with a wide range of impairments of arm function can often manage a vehicle fitted with, for example, ultralight powered steering and various hand and arm steering devices. People who have to remain seated in their wheelchair will need a larger vehicle converted to allow access for the wheelchair to the driving or passenger position. There are a number of specialist conversion companies that can accommodate such needs.

There are very few driving assessment centres. The UK has only around 12 recognized centres and thus many disabled people will have to travel long distances to access such expertise. In the UK there are various government schemes (e.g. Motability) which enable disabled people to use government-backed finance to purchase cars and car adaptations. The community rehabilitation team should certainly be familiar with the broad range of possible adaptations and possibilities and be aware of the nearest driving assessment centre as well as some of the financial funding schemes available to assist disabled people back on to the road.

Having arranged the driving assessment, been deemed fit to drive, and with access to a car with the necessary adaptations, mobility is still not assured. Parking is another problem despite various attempts to rectify the situation such as designated areas for disabled parking. This is echoed in the following comment made by a disabled person: 'Parking is a real problem. There's no good having an 'orange badge' if there's nowhere near your work to park' (Branfield and Maynard Campbell, 2000).

The lack of driving options would be alleviated if access to other forms of transport were made available. Unfortunately this access is notoriously bad. It has been estimated that in Sweden alone, over a million people are unable to use public transport (Iwarsson, 1999). The reasons range from being unreliable, to having restricted wheelchair access and a lack of information about what is available along with the relevant timetables. With insufficient funds to finance alternative means, many disabled people find themselves either dependent on others or unable to travel any substantial distance. This can seriously affect the potential of disabled people to lead full and active lives in their community. Thus efforts to improve access to private or public modes of transport, whether it is a legal requirement or not, are essential.

Education

Return to school or embarking upon tertiary study may be difficult for a number of reasons. Following head injury especially, memory, concentration, processing speed, abstract thinking, attention, energy levels, planning and organizational skills, communication and personality changes may all be affected in some way which will disrupt the educational process. In children, return to school must be carefully planned, and as the demands of the child change so too does the follow-up support (Ponsford et al., 1996). In tertiary education, the demands on a student may be even more pressing due to the structural organization of the working programme and the increasing emphasis placed on self-motivation. Methods to overcome the difficulties associated with continuing education can include ongoing communication between the individual, the family, the original rehabilitation team and a disability liaison officer at the place of education. Any issues may then be dealt with as they arise.

Getting an education is not only important for those with impairments, but it is also true for the rest of society, especially for those working with disability. Education, in the way of disability awareness programmes, can be obtained either as part of standard training procedures or as part of an induction course. It is also imperative to integrate it into the formal training procedures of all health professionals. Attitudes towards disability are still a major obstruction towards the integration of disabled people within community life, thus expanding awareness as part of the school syllabus should be seriously considered.

Psychosocial issues

For those individuals with a severe traumatic brain injury there is a high risk of a significant decline in their friendships and social support, which can result in prolonged loneliness (Morton and Wehman, 1995). The success of transition to independent living in one study was also related to success in developing and maintaining supportive relationships (McColl et al., 1999). It is not only interpersonal relationships with friends, partners and family that impact on community integration, but a diverse range of psychosocial issues. Rehabilitation of young stroke survivors has been associated with a variety of social problems including marital break-up, childcare responsibilities, return to employment, low self-esteem, substance abuse, caregiver-related problems, suicidal tendencies, sexual issues and sexuality, financial concerns, denial, anger, frustration, depression and a return to the parental home (Teasell et al., 2000). There is a need for greater resources to be channelled into psychosocial issues, not just for young people but for all age groups. Furthermore, experience in the field suggests that access to counselling or group therapy to enhance the development of self-awareness, whilst maximizing self-esteem should be provided on an ongoing basis (Ponsford et al., 1996). There is a need for more concrete evidence to support the effectiveness of rehabilitation counselling, otherwise its development within service provision will remain restricted (White and Johnstone, 2000).

Alternative therapies

In a qualitative study that explored the needs of severely disabled people living at home, Stephens found that 'most participants were willing to try new treatments or continue treatments not especially recommended by their doctors in an effort to find alleviation from symptoms. Alternative or complementary treatments featured in many of the participants' decisions' (Stephens, 1998). There are many alternative practices, mainly originating from the South, that are growing in popularity in the North. These include practices such as reflexology, aromatherapy, meditation, yoga, reiki, faith healing and astrology. The use of marijuana is one of the more controversial alternatives, but research studies suggest that it may decrease spasticity and pain (Bowling, 2001). Bowling, although he is specifically referring to MS, promotes an inclusive approach to therapy, which combines conventional therapy with complementary and alternative medicine.

A growing interest in alternative therapies seems to be related to the simultaneous decline of traditional churchgoers. Thus, while it appears that religious belief may be dwindling, people are finding alternative routes through which to find solutions and lead their lives. Hence it would seem only appropriate to acknowledge these interests in the wider picture of holistic rehabilitation. Giving people more choices for treatment that reflect their own lifestyles may be an important ingredient towards gaining empowerment and fulfilment within the rehabilitation process.

Charitable and voluntary agencies

Charitable agencies often follow a traditionally medical model approach to disability. This is evident by the way that they are almost always distinguished according to specific diagnoses. Furthermore, their clients are often portrayed as victims in need of support, which is a direct challenge to the disability movement's drive for equal rights. However, charities are an invaluable resource for many disabled people who would otherwise have little other support. They might be even more effective if they were to work in closer harmony with disability groups and other community services, towards a more consumer-driven focus. Some charities have very high profiles that can attract substantial funds. While this has advantages care must be taken not to lose sight of those in receipt of the benefits.

In the same way, volunteers are a very good source of support. This is especially significant in the South where professionals are in short supply. However, it is important that they are given appropriate training and access to support for themselves.

Legal matters

Many disabled people are involved in litigation, particularly those with cerebral palsy and traumatic brain injury. Litigation in most countries can be a traumatic and stressful process and often prohibitively expensive. The availability of government aid or private insurance varies widely from country to country. The average length of time from initiation of the legal process to final settlement also varies widely but is at least 3 or 4 years in the UK and often longer in cases of cerebral palsy. Eventually a legal settlement for damages can be highly beneficial both for the disabled person and the family. This is particularly so for people with normal expectation of life and an inability to work. Legal settlements can recognize loss of future earnings as well as providing finance for housing and carers. It is not widely known that, at least in the UK, interim settlements are possible for particular expenditures as long as the costs are realistically expected to be within the financial envelope of the final settlement. This can be particularly helpful for purchase of an adapted home or vehicle, for example.

The rather drawn-out legal process can sometimes act as a barrier to rehabilitation. In one study (McColl et al., 1999) it was found that settlement of one participant's insurance claim, and the uncertainties associated with that, acted as a deterrent to the pursuit of rehabilitation.

Financial management is another source of conflict. Clients who are severely impaired may not have the insight and skills to manage their own finances. Issues of consent need to be tackled and further issues may arise over guardianship, marriage and custody. All these factors can have varying and often adverse effects on the community rehabilitation process. It can be a good idea to involve a lawyer as part of the rehabilitation team in order to advise on aspects of care, housing and employment that may be part of a final, and an interim, legal settlement. As always, information and knowledge of the legal process helps to reduce the stress and anxiety associated with it.

Informal care network

We can all give and receive love and we can all care. It seems there is something peculiar in the amount and type of support we give and receive that changes the nature of an (existing) relationship to the type of relationship that is known as 'caregiving' whether the people be spouses, parent, child, friends, or whatever. But where along the continuum of 'the need for support' does the relationship change to be labelled as caregiving rather than being a parent, friend, family or significant person? . . . Is this point called 'disability?'
(Bathurst, 2001)

According to the HACC Legislation and Guidelines in Australia a carer is a 'relative, friend or neighbour who provides unpaid assistance in the activities of daily living to a person who is frail, aged or a younger person with a disability'. There is no doubt that carers (however they may be defined) and families of disabled people are generally expected to shoulder the main burden of care. As described above, caring takes place within an already existing relationship, and the reasons for caring are many (e.g. it may be out of love, duty, or simply a lack of alternatives). Family involvement plays a critical part in stroke rehabilitation (Glass et al., 1992) and the same is likely to be true for other neurological impairments. The question is what aspects of family involvement are critical to successful rehabilitation. Informal care is universally recognized and commonly practised (Ngan and Kwok, 1992) and consequently the literature is fairly extensive. Here, following a look at the epidemiology, the needs of carers will be discussed, followed by an investigation into the support systems available to them and their families. The cultural and political foundations will then be described.

Epidemiology

One in eight people in Britain is now a carer, three-fifths of whom receive no regular visitor support services at all (Department of Health, 1999). One-third of stroke survivors' families describe themselves as not adjusted after 5 years (Holbrook, 1982: cited in Evans et al., 1992). Another study stated that even after 15 years following a traumatic brain injury, the ongoing behavioural effects on the survivors are still having an impact on the caregivers (Frosch et al., 1997). The higher the unmet need of carers the higher their psychiatric morbidity and the lower their quality of life (Moules and Chandler, 1999). One-third of all admissions to a hospital respite programme were directly related to the health of the well spouse (Gaynor, 1990: cited in Holicky, 1996). Similarly, Castree and Barnes (1992) found that 57% of a group of disabled people who had entered institutional care had done so due to their main carer having died (20%) or become unable to cope (37%). The literature documenting the plight of carers is not in short supply, and while it is always necessary to respond to the needs of the disabled people themselves, it is equally important to ensure that their carers are well supported. This not only reduces the vulnerability of carers to psychological and physical ill health, but it also enhances the support system of the disabled person, which is known to boost their own chances of a positive outcome.

Carer needs

There is general consensus about what it is that carers need. Recognition, information, practical help, money, time off, peer support, being valued, being in control and coming to terms with their own feelings summarize the main issues (Pitkeathley, 1991). It is easy to understand that a flexible system is required to respond to individual and unique circumstances especially when the needs of disabled people and their carers will not always be the same. The great variability of experience among carers demands that assessment of needs and planned interventions should be made on an individual basis (Moules and Chandler, 1999).

Arguably the best way in which to appreciate the needs of carers is to listen to what they have to say. While the following extract may appear lengthy it is a raw expression of emotion. It is through its bold directness that Maddison achieves such an eloquent account of her experience as both a carer and a mother:

I realise of course that it is entirely selfish of me to want to resume the 'ordinary' parental role that my peers without disabled offspring enjoy and for my daughter and son to enjoy the benefits of individual choice in lifestyle, that it is selfish of me to want to resume my career, earn a decent wage in order to provide some sort of financial security for myself and my son and daughter, afford the extra costs associated with disability, and Heavens Above perhaps even be indulgent enough to take a day off or a holiday, be spontaneous or be a sexual being . . . You are doing so much for society. You are an enabler – You enable Government to abrogate its responsibility to its citizenry. You are a saver – You lessen the taxpayer burden. You are a contributor – the care role you do saves governments and taxpayers hundreds of thousands of dollars each year. You are a facilitator – the savings you generate facilitate growth in the Human Service sector. You are a role model for industry – it is the work you do that others seek to emulate in paid career opportunities. You are fortunate that you cannot afford alcohol – think of cirrhosis. You are fortunate to be celibate – think AIDS and STDs. You are fortunate that your bills exceed your income – a day of fasting per week is good for body and soul. You are fortunate to feel numb, depressed and have no hope – you will never be disappointed. (Maddison, 2001)

Support systems

Support systems for both families and individual carers vary substantially. They include a range of emotional support, respite, in-home healthcare, information and educational support. Early intervention, especially in the form of assessment and education, are vital. Families also need to be given feedback, and incorporated into the discussion of goals. Often they may find it difficult to come to terms with what has happened, and therefore support groups and family counselling sessions may be useful.

Leach (1996) reported that a family's ability to cope was directly linked to the presence of social support. In another study it was suggested that the more support systems that were reported to be used by caregivers the better able they were to cope with the role changes that occurred (Frosch et al., 1997). Cochran (1994) reported that even just having nurses available to listen and offer some counselling has been useful and successful. Empowerment programmes may also aid families to develop strengths and strategies to face problems. Man (1999) found that an 8-week community-based empowerment programme for a total of 50 family members was found to be effective in improving self-efficacy, broadening knowledge, gaining support and maintaining aspiration.

The benefits of support systems are not always so conclusive. For example, in a study that investigated the impact of social relief admissions, even though they were found to be associated with a definite improvement in mental well-being of caregivers, there was no change in the stress levels reported (Caradoc-Davies and Harvey, 1995). Similarly, in a review of the family's role in stroke rehabilitation, Evans et al. (1992) found that research regarding caregiver support programmes has not succeeded in demonstrating a reduction in subjective burden. Furthermore, the families most in need of supportive care were the least likely to participate.

Cultural and political foundation of informal care

The demand for family support may be dependent on cultural patterns of living. A trend that sees many individuals return to their family home, for example, will increase the stress on carers (Fuentes et al., 1999). Hong Kong has been identified as taking no account of the needs of the caregivers and families of disabled people despite plenty of evidence to suggest that support is required (Kwok, 1995). With decreasing family sizes and a persistent stigma towards the use of nursing homes, families are coming under increasing pressure. There is a strong need to combine informal and formal care to enable families to cope more effectively (Ngan and Kwok, 1992). The lack of a political framework in which to promote such a partnership may be one reason why services for carers and their families are so underdeveloped.

Whatever the cultural background, legislation should enforce that families have access to adequate and appropriate support.

Evidence is emerging to show that effective rehabilitation in the future may be dependent on our ability to understand the dynamics of the family system. There is an intimate link between the family system and the community system, which in turn is linked to national systems, which reinforce the pivotal role of a solid public policy (Frank, 1994). With the growing emphasis on finding cheaper forms of rehabilitative support in the community there is a danger of exploiting family resources. This could lead to a breakdown in the family unit, and subsequent ill health for not only the disabled person but the family members as well. As families and their carers become more involved in the rehabilitation process of the disabled individual, they too will require adequate support mechanisms.

Personal assistants

The experience of caregiving is not always negative. Like any relationship it has positive and negative elements. Berner (1998) became her husband's 'sole caretaker' after he was resuscitated following a cardiac arrest and diagnosed with brain damage. Despite both anger and sadness, she was able to look on the bright side and note that at least now she has more free time to enjoy the better things in life and to spend time with her family after being forced to quit her job. In a study by Johnson (1998) on the positive and negative response to the caregiver role, a sense of loyalty, acceptance, satisfaction and 'feeling good' all emerged from the reports of carers. Even though the benefits of a caring relationship are sparse in the literature, its reciprocal nature is evident. This has been illustrated in the growing rejection of the term itself. There are negative connotations attached to the words 'care' and 'caregiver' in that they imply a one-way relationship with the disabled person being the recipient of help, unable to give anything in return. This has led to the introduction of a new concept; that of a 'personal assistant' or an 'enabler'. By simply employing a different label, it aims to restore the balance of the relationship and shift the control back to the disabled person.

Personal assistants (like 'carers') can assist disabled people in a number of ways to enable them to live at home independently. They can provide assistance in all areas of life depending on the specific requirements of each individual. This can include activities such as personal care, transportation, community access, education, employment, economic security and family life. Personal Assistance Services (PAS) is a system employed in some states of the USA. It evolved from the belief that personal assistance services, with support of the Americans with Disabilities Act, are a human and civil right. Studies across the USA and Europe are showing that many consumers are more satisfied with self-directed personal assistants because it allows them to be in control and have more flexibility (Beatty et al., 1998). Not only are they economically and legally feasible, but research suggests that PAS are linked to increases in work and community engagement (Nosek and Fuhrer, 1995). There is considerable room for development, regarding issues of establishing a cross-disability and cross-age system, that is individualized and has no penalties for working, schooling or marriage (Litvack, 1998).

Personal assistant schemes with a more consumer-driven approach definitely merit closer attention, especially within the political agenda of equalizing the opportunities and rights of disabled people. Increased control and flexibility may not be applicable or desirable for every disabled person. Indeed, many people prefer to relinquish any control and be 'cared' for in the traditional sense. What is of importance is that everyone has the freedom to decide.

Independent living

The concept of 'personal assistants' has developed largely as a result of the independent living movement. Up until recently the lives of disabled people have been largely in the hands of the clinical professions but in reality health is only one part of the picture. The independent living movement thus tends to reflect the aim of this chapter. Independent living (see Chapter 5) developed as a challenge to the medical establishment to enforce the perception that it is disabled people themselves who are the experts in knowing what they want and need; and their needs are not always health-related. Independent living is thus a means for disabled people to access information about all aspects of community life. Advocacy, financial advice, peer support, and access to aids, technology or environmental control systems are all within its repertoire. This makes the independent living movement a critical ally in the drive towards providing more effective rehabilitation.

Conclusion

Medical intervention has dramatically increased the life expectancy of people with impairments but it fails to support and prepare them sufficiently for successful community living after rehabilitation services are terminated (Brandriet et al., 1994). Stroke survivors have emphasized the importance of therapeutic interventions that incorporate people's life interests and goals into the rehabilitation process (Sabari et al., 2000). Although disabled people will always require many forms of medical intervention they cannot be in isolation from other life priorities, such as a house to live in, food to eat and an occupation to provide meaning and identity. Independent living centres tend to better address these issues, taking a more holistic approach.

Limited access to employment, education, transport and leisure facilities hinders the ability of disabled people to exert their independence. The lack of opportunities arise for a number of reasons, including inefficient legislative frameworks. Disabled people often need to sacrifice their independence and rely heavily upon others. Everyone has a unique and complex configuration of experiences and values that constructs their own individual identities. It is important to respect and retain this individuality throughout the rehabilitative process.

Everybody lives within a community and rehabilitation needs to respond to this. It is no longer enough to meet just the health needs of the people who pass through the rehabilitation process. To be truly worthwhile and effective we must encapsulate all the factors that are important to individuals and to do this we need to communicate, learn from and respond at an individual level.

REFERENCES

Allen, L.R. and Beattie, R.J. (1984). The role of leisure as an indicator of overall satisfaction with community life. *Journal of Leisure Research* **2**, 99–109.

Argyle, M. (1967). *The Psychology of Interpersonal Behaviour*. London: Penguin Books.

Barnes, M.P. and Hoyle, E.A. (1995). Driving assessment – a case of need. *Clinical Rehabilitation* **9**, 115–20.

Bathurst, L. (1999). Re: Brain Injury. Disability research mailbase. http://www.mailbase.ac.uk/lists/disability-research/1999-10/0274.html.

Bathurst, L. (2001). Re: The language and baggage of caregiving. Disability research mailbase. http://www.jiscmail.ac.uk/cgi-bin/wa.exe?A2=ind0103andL=disability -researchandP=R5275andm=5471.

Beardshaw, V. (1988). *Last on the List: Community Services for People with Physical Disabilities*. London: King's Fund Institute.

Beatty, P.W., Richmond, G.W., Tepper, S. and DeJong, G. (1998). Personal assistance for people with physical disabilities: consumer-direction and satisfaction with services. *Archives of Physical Medicine and Rehabilitation* **79**, 674–7.

Berner, L.M. (1998). The role of a sole caretaker. *Topics in Stroke Rehabilitation* **5**, 71–2.

Betz, N. and Hackett, G. (1981). The relationship of career related self efficacy expectations to perceived career options in college women and men. *Journal of Counselling Psychology* **28**, 399–410.

Bowling, A.C. (2001). *Alternative Medicine and Multiple Sclerosis*. New York: Demos.

Brandriet, L.M., Lyons, M. and Bentley, J. (1994). Perceived needs of poststroke elders following termination of home health services. *Nursing and Health Care* **15**, 514–20.

Branfield, F. and Maynard Campbell, S. (2000). *Common Barriers and their Removal – Report of Research into Barriers to Employment and Training Faced by Disabled People and their Employers and Training Providers*. Manchester: Breakthrough UK Ltd.

Caradoc-Davies, T.H. and Harvey, J.M. (1995). Do 'social relief' admissions have any effect on patients or their care-givers? *Disability and Rehabilitation* **17**, 247–51.

Castree, B.J. and Barnes, M.P. (1992). Informal care networks – One of the keys to community care. *Clinical Rehabilitation* **6** (Suppl.), 40–1.

Chawla, J.C. (1994). Sport for people with disability. *British Medical Journal* **308**, 1500–4.

Christensen, A. (1992). Outpatient management and outcome in relation to work in traumatic brain injury patients. *Scandinavian Journal of Rehabilitation Medicine* **Suppl. 26**, 34–42.

Cochran, J. (1994). Family caregivers of the frail elderly: burdens and health. *Nurse Practitioner* **91**, 5–6.

Department of Health (1999). Caring About Carers: A National Strategy for Carers. http://www.doh.gov.uk/carers.htm.

Devlieger, P.J. (1999). From handicap to disability: language use and cultural meaning in the United States. *Disability and Rehabilitation* **21**, 346–54.

Drummond, A.E.R. and Walker, M.F. (1994). The Nottingham Leisure Questionnaire for stroke patients. *British Journal of Occupational Therapy* **57**, 414–18.

Drummond, A.E.R. and Walker, M.F. (1996). Generalisation of the effects of leisure rehabilitation for stroke patients. *British Journal of Occupational Therapy* **59**, 330–4.

Duckett, P.S. (2000). Disabling employment interviews: warfare to work. *Disability and Society* **15**, 1019–39.

Dunn, P.A. (1990). The impact of the housing environment upon the ability of disabled people to live independently. *Disability, Handicap and Society* **5**, 37.

Evans, R.L., Hendricks, R.D., Haselkorn, J.K. et al. (1992). The family's role in stroke rehabilitation: a review of the literature. *American Journal of Physical Medicine and Rehabilitation* **71**, 135–9.

Fange, A. and Iwarsson, S. (1999). Physical housing environment: development of a self-assessment instrument. *Canadian Journal of Occupational Therapy* **66**, 250–60.

Floyd, M. (1991). Overcoming barriers to employment. In *Disability and Social Policy*, ed. G. Dalley. London: PSI Publication.

Fox, G.K., Bowden, S.C. and Smith, D.S. (1998). On-road assessment of driving competence after brain impairment: review of current practice and recommendations for a standardised examination. *Archives of Physical Medicine and Rehabilitation* **79**, 1288–96.

Frank, R.G. (1994). Families and rehabilitation. *Brain Injury* **8**, 193–5.

Frosch, S., Gruber, A., Jones, C. et al. (1997). The long term effects of traumatic brain injury on the roles of caregivers. *Brain Injury* **11**, 891–906.

Fuentes, M.G., Baker, J.G., Markello, S.J. and Wood, K.D. (1999). Discharge to home among Hispanic and non-Hispanic stroke survivors: does family make a difference? *International Journal of Rehabilitation Research* **22**, 317–20.

Glass, T.A., Matchar, D.B., Belyea, M. and Feussner, J.R. (1992). Impact of social support on outcome in first stroke. *Stroke* **24**, 64–70.

Gouvier, W.D. and Steiner, D.D. (1991). Employment discrimination against handicapped job candidates: an analog study of the effects of neurological causation, visibility of handicap, and public contact. *Rehabilitation Psychology* **36**, 121–9.

Heller, T., Factor, A.R. and Hahn, J. E. (1999). Residential transitions from nursing homes for adults with cerebral palsy. *Disability and Rehabilitation* **21**, 277–83.

Holicky, R. (1996). Caring for the caregivers: the hidden victims of illness and disability. *Rehabilitation Nursing* **21**, 247–52.

Iwarsson, S. (1999). The housing enabler: an objective tool for accessing accessibility. *British Journal of Occupational Therapy* **62**, 491–7.

Iwarsson, S. and Isacsson, A. (1996). Development of a novel instrument for occupational therapy assessment of the physical environment in the home – a methodological study on 'The Enabler'. *Occupational Therapy Journal of Research* **16**, 227–44.

Iwarsson, S. and Isacsson, A. (1997). Quality of life in the elderly population: an example exploring interrelationships among subjective well-being, ADL dependence, and housing accessibility. *Archives of Gerontology and Geriatrics* **26**, 71–83.

Jackson, J.D. (1994). After rehabilitation: meeting the long-term needs of persons with traumatic brain injury. *American Journal of Occupational Therapy* **48**, 251–5.

Johnson, P.D. (1998). Rural stroke caregivers: a qualitative study of the positive and negative response to the caregiver role. *Topics in Stroke Rehabilitation* **5**, 51–68.

Johnson, R. (1987). Return to work after severe head injury. *Disability Studies* **9**, 49–54.

Knobbe, C.A., Carey, S.P., Rhodes, L. and Horner, R.H. (1995). Benefit-cost analysis of community residential versus institutional services for adults with severe mental retardation and challenging behaviors. *American Journal of Mental Retardation* **99**, 533–41.

Kwok, J. (1995). The role of the family in disability concerned policies and services: challenges for community based rehabilitation in the Asian and Pacific decade of disabled persons, 1993–2002. *International Journal of Rehabilitation Research* **18**, 351–6.

Leach, B. (1996). Disabled people and the equal opportunities movement. In *Beyond Disability: Towards an Enabling Society*, ed. G. Hales, pp. 88–95. Bristol, PA: The Open University.

Litvak, S. (1998). Personal assistance services policy: where we have been and where are we going. *American Rehabilitation* **24**, 9–14.

Lougheed, V. (1998). Employer-based rehabilitation. *Canadian Journal of Rehabilitation* **12**, 33–7.

Maddison, F. (2001). Re: The language and baggage of caregiving. Disability research mailbase. http://www.jiscmail.ac.uk/cgi-bin/wa.exe?A2=ind0103andL=disability-researchandP=R7321andm=5471.

Man, D. (1999). Community-based empowerment programme for families with a brain injured survivor: an outcome study. *Brain Injury* **13**, 433–45.

Mank, D., Cioffi, A. and Yovanoff, P. (1997). Patterns of support for employees with severe disabilities. *Mental Retardation.* **35**, 433–47.

McColl, M.A., Davies, D., Carlson, P. et al. (1999). Transitions to independent living after ABI. *Brain Injury* **13**, 311–30.

Morton, M.V. and Wehman, P. (1995). Psychosocial and emotional sequelae of individuals with traumatic brain injury: a literature review and recommendations. *Brain Injury* **9**, 81–92.

Moules, S. and Chandler, B.J. (1999). A study of the health and social needs of carers of traumatically brain injured individuals served by one community rehabilitation team. *Brain Injury* **13**, 983–93.

Ngan, R. and Kwok, J. (1992). Informal caring networks among Chinese elderly with disabilities in Hong Kong. *International Journal of Rehabilitation Research* **15**, 199–207.

Nosek, M. and Fuhrer, M. (1995). Life satisfaction of people with physical disabilities: relationship to personal assistance, disability status, and handicap. *Rehabilitation Psychology* **40**, 191–202.

Parker, C.J., Gladman, J.R.F. and Drummond, A.E.R. (1997). The role of leisure in stroke rehabilitation. *Disability and Rehabilitation* **19**, 1–5.

Parker, C.J., Gladman, J.R.F., Drummond, A.E.R. et al. (2001). A multicentre randomized controlled trial of leisure therapy and conventional occupational therapy after stroke. *Clinical Rehabilitation* **15**, 42–52.

Partners in Policy making (1993). Curriculum highlights – Topic 4: Supported, competitive employment. http://www.partnersinpolicymaking.com/curriculum/Topic4.htm.

Perino, C., Zappala, G., Verne, D. and Rago, R. (2000). Neuropsychological rehabilitation and return to work after TBI: an Italian experience. *Brain Injury Source* **4**, http://www.biausa.org/bis_vol4issue2.htm.

Pitkeathley, J. (1991). The carers' viewpoint. In *Disability and Social Policy*, ed. G. Dalley, pp. 203–9. London: PSI Publication.

Ponsford, J., Sloan, S. and Snow, P. (1996). *Traumatic Brain Injury – Rehabilitation for Everyday Adaptive Living.* Hove: Psychology Press.

Sabari, J.S., Meisler, J. and Silver, E. (2000). Reflections upon rehabilitation by members of a community based stroke club. *Disability and Rehabilitation* **22**, 330–6.

Soderback, I., Ekholm, J. and Caneman, G. (1991). Impairment/function and disability/activity 3 years after cerebrovascular incident or brain trauma: a rehabilitation and occupational therapy view. *International Disability Studies* **13**, 67–73.

Soderback, I., Pekkanen, K., Ekholm, J. and Schuldt, K. (1993). Occupational therapy work training programs for brain-damaged individuals – A Swedish program. *Work* **3**, 37–47.

Stephens, J. (1998). The needs of severely disabled people living at home: how do severely disabled people living at home manage their health care needs? *Action Aid Disability News* **9**, 51–5.

Teasell, R.W., McRae, M.P. and Finestone, H.M. (2000). Social issues in the rehabilitation of younger stroke patients. *Archives of Physical Medicine and Rehabilitation* **81**, 205–9.

Trach, J.S. and Shelden, D.L. (1999). Natural supports as a foundation for support-based employment development and facilitation. *American Rehabilitation* **25**, 2–7.

van Lierop, B. and Nijhuis, F. (2000). Assessment, education and placement: an integrated approach to vocational rehabilitation. *International Journal of Rehabilitation Research* **23**, 261–9.

van Zomeren, A.H., Brouwer, W.H. and Minderhoud, J.M. (1987). Acquired brain damage and driving: a review. *Archives of Physical Medicine and Rehabilitation* **68**, 697–705.

Wehman, P. and Revell, G. (1998). Supported employment: a decade of rapid growth and impact. *American Rehabilitation* **24**, 31–43.

White, M.A. and Johnstone, A.S. (2000). Recovery from stroke: does rehabilitation counselling have a role to play? *Disability and Rehabilitation* **22**, 140–3.

10

Community rehabilitation in childhood: concepts to inform practice

Peter Rosenbaum and Mary Law

McMaster University, Hamilton, Ontario

Introduction

Jenna is a 6-year-old girl, the second of two children of a mother who is 29 and her 32-year-old husband. Jenna was born unexpectedly at 30 weeks gestation following an uneventful pregnancy, and experienced a variety of perinatal difficulties requiring a stay in the special care baby unit. Following discharge she was seen regularly at a newborn follow-up clinic, where her developmental progress was monitored carefully. At 8 months Jenna's motor development was 'slow' and she appeared somewhat 'stiff'. At 1 year of age, adjusting for her prematurity, she was thought to have 'cerebral palsy', the prognosis of which was uncertain. At 2 years her language was 'delayed', but at 3 she had caught up with speech. She entered school at the usual age but needed special help with mobility, and some extra attention for her learning. Throughout this period from birth to age 6 Jenna's family saw a succession of professionals, received extensive but at times conflicting information and advice, and sought the latest news about therapies from the internet.

How might one approach the 'rehabilitation' needs of Jenna and her family? What are realistic goals, and how should they be achieved? What is Jenna's prognosis, and on what evidence is any judgement based?

To understand the 'rehabilitation' of children with disabilities professionals need to be familiar with several conceptual underpinnings that distinguish children's needs from those of adults. The purpose of this chapter is to outline and explain these concepts. We believe that it is essential to recognize the special elements of childhood that influence what is done with children, in what ways, with whom and for what reasons. The emphases are therefore more on process and rationale than on specific content of childhood rehabilitation, though examples from the field of paediatric rehabilitation will be used throughout to illustrate the points that are presented. At the end of the chapter we shall return to offer some thoughts about how Jenna and her family might be well served by the service providers and community agencies whose roles are important for Jenna's well-being.

Childhood disability

What do we mean by 'childhood disability'? The following definition was created recently by a group of Canadian rehabilitation professionals, parents and policy makers who attended a conference on research issues in the field of childhood disability. Inherent in the definition are the key elements that will form the substance of this chapter.

Childhood disabilities refer to differences in children's development or current functioning (in any or all of the spheres of physical, cognitive, affective, social, communicative, or sensory function) resulting from interactions of conditions that are intrinsic to the child, and environmental factors which may present barriers to full development and function. Such conditions (intrinsic) and the interactions of these within environmental settings, including societal attitudes and values (extrinsic), present special challenges for the child and their family, as well as for institutional systems, communities, and future employers.

By definition, childhood disability may present a constantly changing picture, with new outcomes emerging from old. Throughout their growing years children are by nature in a state of change and development; hence disorders of development may have diverse and cumulative impacts on many aspects of a child's development and function as the child grows. Similarly, children's and families' needs change constantly throughout childhood and adolescence. Supports and services, as well as research, must be designed and constructed in a manner that is sensitive to and addresses these issues so that full inclusion and participation of children with disabilities is possible. (*CanChild* Centre for Childhood Disability Research).

The central element in all considerations about children is the fact that they are in a constant state of 'becoming'. That is, they (and their conditions) are developing and changing in ways that are profoundly important to their well-being, and which clearly must be considered when one is offering any type of rehabilitative services. Of paramount importance to the child is the *impact* of any condition or disorder – be it congenital or acquired – on the child's development. This point is important because conditions that restrict a child's capacities in any way may influence the trajectory of their development. The corollary of this perspective is that interventions that enhance a child's functional capabilities may have a very important effect in moderating the impact of the impairments that underlie any developmental disorder. We shall return to this idea later in the chapter.

The 'ecology' of childhood

It is essential to start by stating a truism about children – namely that they grow and develop within an 'ecological' context of family and community. One must therefore recognize the role and influence of family as integral to whatever services are offered to children, and to acknowledge the primacy of the roles of parents in decision-making about their child's rehabilitation. In many places the concepts of 'family-centred services' have been articulated and adopted as guides to the style, process and content of rehabilitation services (King et al., 1998; Rosenbaum et al., 1998). Research evidence shows that there is a direct and important link between parents' experiences of the family-centredness of their child's care and their satisfaction, the stress they experience with these services and their mental health (King S et al., 1996; King et al., 1999). Therefore if one believes that the well-being of children is enhanced by the quality of their parents' lives, service provision will be organized and delivered in ways that minimize parental distress and recognize the family as the unit of interest in childhood rehabilitation.

Equally important is the influence of the 'community' in which child and family live, since it is community players (such as nurseries, schools, recreational programmes, social services and other public as well as private agencies (e.g. insurance companies)) that may play a determining role in enabling or preventing full participation of children with disabilities in the life of their community (Law et al., 1999). As will be discussed later, current World Health Organization concepts talk of 'participation' as the ultimate goal of health, and thus of successful rehabilitation (WHO, 2001). It is therefore essential that a child's rehabilitation takes place within a community context of school, recreational programmes, public facilities etc., and that efforts be directed at the environments in which a child might wish or need to function. The concept of the integration of 'person–environment–occupation' has received much attention in the field of occupational therapy (Law et al., 1996) and is increasingly being seen as a way to broaden the scope of services for people with disabilities. The success of a person in performing daily life activities is the direct result of many complex interactions between that person, the activities they choose to do and the environment in which the activities are carried out.

Child development as an organizing principle

It may seem self-evident that children are in a constant state of development and change. It is however important to reiterate the obvious in order to place in context the principles by which developmental rehabilitation is provided. First, one must consider the age and stage of each child when assessing development and function, and in planning interventions. Both the functional capacity and the emerging skills of children are strongly age-dependent. Furthermore, the capacities of children can vary across dimensions of development. For example, two children of the same age with cerebral palsy of similar severity might have very different needs based on factors such as visual or cognitive impairments. Therapy services must therefore be tailored to each child's developmental abilities in many dimensions of function, as well as their chronological age.

A second 'developmental' implication of developmental disabilities concerns the *impact* of a disability on a child's overall development. Consider as an example a preschool child with a developmental motor problem (though the same arguments, by analogy, can be made if a child has sensory, cognitive or language disability). The effect of restricted mobility experience on a child's overall development can be significant – for example, by limiting exploration of space and thereby impeding the neuromotor learning associated with movement. A child with limited capacity to move independently may be inhibited in their opportunities to practice new skills repeatedly (as typically occurs throughout childhood), in turn limiting the child's experiences of the social consequences (both positive and negative) of motor activities such as touching things, running to and away from people, and exploring in ways that parents don't allow! To the extent that disability limits typical childhood experiences, a child with a disability can often be thought of as a child growing up 'deprived'. These considerations certainly have implications for planning interventions.

When one considers the enormous variability among children and families, and the variations in child-rearing practices within a community, let alone across cultures, it becomes apparent that there is no single route to successful development. We believe that it is not helpful to talk of 'normal' and 'abnormal' development, with the implication that these apparent distinctions are meaningful and mutually exclusive categories into which children's development can be placed. Rather one should look at the individual predicament (Taylor, 1982) of each child with a disability and consider whether, and in what ways, the presence of a biopsychosocial impairment does or potentially might influence developmental trajectories. If the goal of childhood is to emerge at the end of the first 20 years of life as a capable, competent, confident young adult with as much independence as possible, one's 'interventions' during childhood for children with 'disabilities' take on a focus that promotes these characteristics and abilities rather than addressing 'abnormality' ('impairment' in WHO (2001) terms) in the traditional biomedical sense, and trying to 'fix' them.

This last idea points to the need to recognize that developmental rehabilitation cannot be seen simply as a series of events and 'treatments'. It is rather a process that aims to promote the best development of each child under the circumstances of their impairments, in the context of their abilities, their family and their community. This thinking reflects a shift in focus from the biomedical approach toward the broader WHO (2001) emphasis on 'activity' and 'participation' as the goals of life – goals we believe can be successfully incorporated into the rehabilitation programmes of children with disabilities.

The challenges and limitations of 'diagnosis'

In the medical field diagnosis has traditionally been seen as an essential point for initiation of intervention. This is most obviously true in acute care situations, in which an accurate diagnosis leads to specific courses of action, and where erroneous formulations about a condition may misguide therapeutic efforts. Furthermore one often seeks to 'rule out' competing diagnostic possibilities toward the identification of the 'right' diagnosis. This approach is clearly important in all areas of clinical practice, but may by itself have limited utility and cause some restrictions on thinking and therefore on rehabilitation practice. It is important to explore these ideas in the context of childhood disability.

Many of the 'diagnoses' associated with childhood disabilities – terms like 'cerebral palsy', 'pervasive developmental disorder/autism' or 'mental retardation' – are in fact 'conditions' defined phenomenologically rather than 'diseases' that can consistently be described in biological terms. That is to say, they represent the phenotypic manifestations of a host of underlying biological impairments that are sometimes, but not always, found to be associated with the clinical 'syndromes' that we call, for example, cerebral palsy, autism or mental retardation. (In fact there are still a large proportion of cases in which even with clear evidence of developmental disability one is at a loss to identify the biological basis of the condition.)

Thus more often than not while the 'diagnosis' can provide information about the types of developmental and functional impacts of that condition on a child, it leaves much more to be ascertained through a careful look at the individual. As an example, children with the 'cerebral palsies' have, by definition, '. . . non-progressive, but often changing, motor impairment syndromes secondary to lesions or anomalies of the brain arising in the early stages of development' (Mutch et al., 1992). The hallmark of the cerebral palsies is an impairment in the development of motor control and posture. Any impairment in brain structure causing developmental motor limitations is likely often to be associated with other CNS-related functional consequences that are frequent, but not invariable, comorbidities of 'cerebral palsy'. The 'diagnosis' of cerebral palsy by itself therefore provides quite limited information, and certainly conveys no ideas about the nature, severity, or distribution of the motor difficulties, let alone about any associated conditions.

Another complexity associated with making a diagnosis of developmental disabilities is the issue of when one can be confident about making a diagnosis at all! This occurs because apart from acquired conditions associated with a discrete event (such as trauma) most developmental disabilities emerge over time against a background of expected development. In these situations it is the failure of typical milestones or behaviours to appear at an age-appropriate stage that provides a first signal that there may be difficulties with a child's development. Even here however one must consider whether one is observing a variation of patterns of typical development as opposed to an 'abnormal' trajectory requiring intervention. This is true of variations in motor, language, social and cognitive development, and makes the issue of 'diagnosis' of a 'condition' sometimes quite challenging. Furthermore, simply by virtue of the patterns of child development, delay in one area of development may become evident long before problems in another area are apparent.

For example, gross motor delay may be seen in a child who later turns out to have features of pervasive developmental disorder (PDD). At 10 or 12 months these motor delays may not (yet) be associated with the impairments in language and social development or the behavioural characteristics that are the hallmarks of PDD in a child over the age of 3 years. The 'diagnosis' here may not be apparent for many months, and will depend upon a careful assessment and close follow-up to evaluate the emerging clinical picture. This example also illustrates the potential perils of making an early definitive diagnosis, with its attendant prognosis and approaches to intervention, when the story has not developed far enough for one to be certain.

It is always important to have in mind a differential set of considerations about 'diagnosis' and how best to formulate what is actually interfering with a child's progress. Consider for example a child at age 2 with what seems to be delayed language development. That child might have any – or indeed all – of several problems. The child may have hearing difficulties that interfere with language acquisition. There may be parenting problems, which result in neglect and failure of the parents to provide the adequate language modelling essential to language development. If the child also has 'intrinsic' limitations in cognitive capability, the impact of these other factors will be multiplicative rather than additive. Under these circumstances, to name but four of several, that child may appear 'autistic', 'retarded', 'language impaired', 'hearing impaired' or perhaps all of the above. The assessment of such problems therefore must be undertaken thoughtfully in order to 'rule in' all the elements that could be contributing to the clinical picture of developmental disability, rather than trying to make a specific diagnosis with the implication that if the child has 'this' disorder they cannot have 'that' one.

The locus of interventions

From what has been said thus far it must be apparent that for the vast majority of children with disabilities rehabilitation takes place outside of a hospital setting, and outside the frameworks of conventional medicine. Children with disabilities and their families live at home and function in the community, and it is to these venues that services should be directed. We alluded earlier in this chapter to the importance of recognizing not only the person with the disability, but also the environments in which they function and the tasks that are important to them. In this model the environments in which children live and function become an important target of intervention activity, as are efforts to ensure an appropriate fit between child and task. Thus in addition to the specific technical services provided by developmental professionals, there is an important role for partnerships with parents, as well as for advocacy, community education, community development and environmental 'engineering'. All these efforts will be directed toward facilitating activity and participation for children whose functional needs may make 'ordinary' involvement in their community more difficult than usual.

Emerging concepts of dynamic systems theory, methods of caregiving and family-centred service, are beginning to prompt therapists to consider alternative ways of conceptualizing motor development and intervention for children (Dunst et al., 1988; Darrah et al., 2001). In contrast to the hierarchical model of neural organization, dynamic systems theory posits a flexible model of neural organization in which the functions of control and coordination are distributed among many elements of the system rather than vested in a single hierarchical level (Van Sant, 1991). Dynamic systems theory views motor behaviour as emerging from the dynamic cooperation of the many subsystems in a task-specific context.

In dynamic systems theory, three major components help or hinder completion of a motor behaviour: the child, the environment and the targeted activity/task. To learn new movements or ways of completing an activity, previously stable movements break down or become unstable. New movements and skills emerge when there is a critical change in any of the components, which contribute to motor behaviour. These periods of change are called *transitions*. Motor change in young children is envisioned as a series of events during which destabilizing and stabilizing of movement take place before a transitional phase movement becomes stable and functional.

The ideas from dynamic systems theory, along with the emerging emphasis on parent involvement in therapy, converge toward the development of a family-centred functional intervention approach for children with neurological problems (Law et al., 1998). Within this approach, the emphasis in therapy is on promotion of function through identifying tasks/skills in transition, and identifying and changing constraints to performance of these tasks.

The challenges inherent in this model will be obvious. They include the need to 'educate' people in the community who are responsible for children's activities, such as teachers, recreational specialists and 'adult'-oriented health professionals, to the special needs of children and families where disability is part of the child's life. For many people unfamiliar with concepts such as the ones being raised here, it is too easy to want to 'fix' the child with 'therapy', rather than adapt the tasks and environments to accommodate the abilities as well as the functional needs of the child. It has been our experience that many professionals familiar mainly with typical children, and certainly most professionals who work with adults, will simply be unaware of the concepts that are being outlined here. It is for this reason that 'education' and advocacy on behalf of children with disabilities, and their families, is so important.

This last point identifies the requirement for child-oriented rehabilitation professionals to spend much of their time as advocates, educators and activists on behalf of their clients, explaining the ways in which children's disabilities and rehabilitation differ from the needs and services for adults and those of typically developing children. It is essential that people understand that children are not small adults, but have distinct needs of their own both by virtue of their stage in life and because of the implications of disability on development. For example, an orthopaedist who works primarily with adults may not be as aware of the developmental changes that occur in the bones and joints of a small child, let alone in the natural developmental changes in function, that characterize children's progress through the developing years. As a consequence they may want to intervene 'aggressively', perhaps to align a limb surgically or alter muscle pulls around a joint. In contrast, a specialist with training and experience with children might bring a perspective about the potential changeability of children's structure and function with less active intervention or perhaps simply through developmental change.

Ways of being helpful — what do parents want from professionals?

In the context of the model of family-centred services referred to earlier professionals need to recognize the family as the unit of interest when planning and providing services for a child with a disability. Research evidence points clearly to the need identified by parents for information, for continuity and consistency in service provision, for partnerships with the professionals working with them and their child and for respectful and supportive care (Rosenbaum et al., 1992). By accepting the 'noncategorical' view of chronic childhood conditions (Pless and Pinkerton, 1975), which posits that the common elements across disorders have much in common despite the biological diversity of various conditions, it becomes obvious that these elements are no less important to families of children with long-term problems of health, such as cystic fibrosis and diabetes mellitus (Baine et al., 1995).

These considerations have importance when it comes to the models of service organization by which a developmental programme is provided (Robards, 1994). Families want and need consistency and continuity from the professionals with whom they work, and find the discontinuities common to many university-affiliated programmes quite frustrating (Breslau and Mortimer, 1981). Interestingly, as Breslau showed in subsequent work (1982), continuity is of much greater importance to parents of children with chronic than with episodic healthcare needs. Thus one implication of the way that services are provided is that there need to be people staffing the service who represent familiar faces and voices to families from one clinic encounter to the next. This seems to be important in order for families to be able to pick up where they left off at the last visit, rather than starting again with new people. The continuity staff may be medical personnel, but equally helpful are people who fulfil a clinic 'coordinator' role and who know the families and their issues. The professional discipline of these coordinators is probably less important than the functional roles they provide, though by their professional experience community-oriented nurses or social workers often seem especially well suited to the role of liaison between the family and the rest of the clinical team.

A model that, in our opinion, is less effective is the 'assessment clinic' approach where a child is seen for a consultation opinion, but where there is no planned continuing connection with the child and family. From the family's perspective the potential limitations of this model include the lack of follow-up with the people who have made an initial formulation about their child (Rosenbaum, 1988). Thus it may be difficult for the family to revisit issues with the people they saw originally if these questions occur to the family after they have left the assessment clinic. For the professionals in an assessment clinic model there is no opportunity either to reassess the child and family some time later, when the clinical story and findings may have evolved, or to evaluate (and learn about) the progress a child and family will make over time. The professionals' knowledge about child development will therefore be based largely on cross-sectional assessment experience rather than the longitudinal perspectives gleaned from seeing the same children and families at different times in their development. This consideration is especially vital for learners who need to become aware of possibilities for child and family resilience after the initial diagnosis of a developmental disability, which may cause great distress to a family.

Is there evidence that any of this really matters to families? Work in family-centred services has shown that there are strong correlations between parents' experience of the family-centredness of the services they receive and their overall satisfaction and the stress they perceive in their dealings with their child's professionals (King S et al., 1996). Evidence drawn largely from the adult literature shows that satisfaction, stress and adherence to therapy recommendations are all correlated with the provision of the quality of the services (King G et al., 1996). The qualities that have been described include, not surprisingly, provision of information, respectful services and partnership/enabling. Furthermore there is recent evidence of a modest but significant connection between the family-centredness of services and parental mental health (King et al., 1999). Thus for professionals concerned with family well-being the nature and organization of services for children with developmental disabilities really does matter to families. If one needs a reason to address parents' and families' as well as children's issues, this focus can be considered an important element in the prevention of secondary stress and mental health problems in parents of these children, whose lives are known to be more stressed than the lives of families of well children (Cadman et al., 1991).

Studies repeatedly identify parents' need for information about their child and their condition. It is necessary to say a word about the universal availability of information through the internet, and the challenge that this poses for both consumers and professionals. The internet promotes the free exchange of ideas, and often seems to be a valuable source of contacts for people with similar predicaments. At the same time, as a relatively unregulated information source, there is often material available that has not stood the conventional test of peer review, and at times may be frankly wrong. Furthermore, promoters of various 'treatments' – both conventional and 'alternative' therapies – appear to be relying ever more heavily on the internet to sell their ideas.

The implications of the information explosion for parents include the possibility that they or their friends will hear about new and promising ideas apparently relevant to the needs of their child – often before conventional practitioners! They then may seek our advice about interventions about which they are better informed than their service providers. We believe (Rosenbaum, 1997) that a frank and honest discussion about complementary and alternative therapies is usually helpful to families. Some will pursue every avenue while others will elect to trust the judgement of their providers and wait for stronger evidence than is usually available about innovative 'breakthroughs', particularly those driven by a profit motive.

Long-term planning of intervention for Jenna and her family

Returning to Jenna, what service provision scenario might one have painted for her family from the time she was born, and certainly from the time when there were first concerns about her development?

In an ideal world, when there were concerns about her development, Jenna and her family would be referred to a speciality children's developmental rehabilitation programme, perhaps a regional centre such as those described for the UK setting by Robards (1994). There they would be seen by service providers with experience and expertise in what we refer to as 'applied child development' – an understanding of the nature and impact of childhood disability on the development of children and their families. Counselling would include appropriate 'truth disclosure' about Jenna's situation, with time for discussion and reflection by both the family and the professionals (Cunningham et al., 1984). To the extent that her parents asked about prognosis ('How bad is it?' 'Will Jenna walk on her own?'), they could be counselled about ways of describing the 'severity' of Jenna's cerebral palsy (Palisano et al., 1997) and the probability that she would become independent in her mobility (Palisano et al., 2000).

Subsequently family and professionals would plan Jenna's 'developmental rehabilitation' programme together. Shared goal-setting would emerge from discussions in which professionals outline options for intervention and the family contributes to the planning, to the extent that they feel comfortable to do so. The team working with Jenna would communicate with each other and a 'prime therapist' or other 'lead' professional would be the family's main connection with the 'system'. Continuity of providers over time would be an important goal of the programme, with the family having the option as to whom they felt most comfortable to work with.

In addition to the developmental, therapy and technical interventions that Jenna might receive it would be important for everyone involved with her – family and professionals alike – to reassess her developmental progress and emerging needs on at least an annual basis. The perspectives provided by such a review enable everyone concerned to annotate (and perhaps measure formally) Jenna's progress. This has both important psychological value for her family (and the professionals) and forms the basis for a reformulation of goals related to changing abilities and new developmental capabilities.

As Jenna's horizons expand beyond immediate family to nursery or pre-school, it would be important to help her parents find programmes that are sensitive to the needs and capacity of children with developmental disabilities. Advocacy on behalf of child and family are often needed, in the form of letters of introduction, visits to community-based facilities, provision of reading materials about a child's disability, and so on. Often agencies such as insurance companies, familiar with adult disability claims, require a lay version of the child's story and an explanation of why, for example, it might be very appropriate to prescribe a powered mobility aid for a 3-year old.

Challenges and unmet needs for Jenna and her family

There are a number of areas where there remains little systematic experience and few guidelines for the provision of services to children and youth with developmental disabilities. As Jenna moves into the adolescent years her needs will change both in terms of typical developmental stages and in relation to the impact of her developmental differences. Few developmental disability programmes provide ongoing developmental and health surveillance for young people at this stage of life; nor are adult-oriented services generally equipped to address the needs of people who have grown up with developmental disabilities. Families describe the metaphor of 'falling off the cliff' at the end of childhood (Stewart, 1998), and of subsequently feeling abandoned by the systems which at their best had supported them through their child's early years. This will be a very real challenge for Jenna's family.

It is apparent that one of the major issues to be addressed by both child-focused and adult rehabilitation services are ways to develop seamless transitions across these programmes. To accomplish this will require the integration of both professional activities and conceptual frameworks, with each group learning to understand the perspectives of the other. It is essential that professionals working with children with disabilities and their families know what will be available to these young people in their adult years, and that they strive to prepare them for the 'adult' world to which they are heading. It is equally important to learn lessons from adults with developmental disabilities in order to feed these perspectives back to those who work with children and families. It is vital for people whose thinking is 'developmental' to share this orientation with professionals working to 'rehabilitate' adults back to a state of previous health and function – an orientation substantially different from the 'developmental' perspectives of people working in developmental rehabilitation.

The world in which Jenna and her family are growing up is far more receptive and attuned to their needs than it would have been 25 years ago. However, much remains to be accomplished if we are to be able to support the development and full self-actualization of young people with developmental disabilities. Opportunities abound, and the payoff to the whole community will be well worth the effort.

REFERENCES

Baine, S., Rosenbaum, P. and King, S. (1995). Chronic childhood illnesses: what aspects of caregiving do parents value? *Child: Care, Health and Development* **21**, 291–304.

Breslau, N. (1982). Continuity re-examined: differential impact on satisfaction with medical care for disabled and normal children. *Medical Care* **XX**, 347–60.

Breslau, N. and Mortimer, E.A. (1981). Seeing the same doctor: determinants of satisfaction with specialty care for disabled children. *Medical Care* **XIX**, 741–57.

Cadman, D., Rosenbaum, P., Boyle, M. and Offord, D.R. (1991). Children with chronic illness: family and parent demographic characteristics and psychosocial adjustment. *Pediatrics* **87**, 884–9.

CanChild: www.fhs.mcmaster.ca/canchild/.

Cunningham, C.C., Morgan, P.A. and McGucken, R.B. (1984). Down's syndrome: is dissatisfaction with disclosure of diagnosis inevitable? *Developmental Medicine and Child Neurology* **26**, 33–9.

Darrah, J., Law, M. and Pollock, N. (2001). Family-centred functional therapy. A choice for children with motor dysfunction. *Infants and Young Children* **13**, 79–87.

Dunst, C., Trivette, C. and Deal, A. (1988). *Enabling and Empowering Families – Principles and Guidelines for Practice*. Cambridge, MA: Brookline Books.

King, G., King, S. and Rosenbaum, P. (1996). Interpersonal aspects of caregiving and client outcomes: a review of the literature. *Ambulatory Child Health* **2**, 151–60.

King, G., Law, M., King, S. and Rosenbaum, P. (1998). Parents' and service providers' perceptions of the family-centredness of children's rehabilitation services in Ontario. *Physical and Occupational Therapy in Pediatrics* **18**, 21–40.

King, G., King, S., Rosenbaum, P. and Goffin, R. (1999). Family-centred caregiving and well-being of parents of children with disabilities: linking process with outcome! *Journal of Pediatric Psychology* **24**, 41–52.

King, S., Rosenbaum, P. and King, G. (1996). Parents' perceptions of care-giving: development and validation of a process measure. *Developmental Medicine and Child Neurology* **38**, 757–72.

Law, M., Cooper, B.A., Strong, S. et al. (1996). The person-environment-occupation model: a transactive approach to occupational therapy. *Canadian Journal of Occupational Therapy* **63**, 9–23.

Law, M., Darrah, J., Rosenbaum, P. et al. (1998). Family-centred functional therapy for children with cerebral palsy: an emerging practice model. *Physical and Occupational Therapy in Pediatrics* **18**, 83–102.

Law, M., Haight, M., Milroy, B. et al. (1999). Environmental factors affecting the occupations of children with physical disabilities. *Journal of Occupational Science* **6**, 102–10.

Mutch, L., Alberman, E., Hagberg, B. et al. (1992). Cerebral palsy epidemiology: where are we now and where are we going? *Developmental Medicine and Child Neurology* **34**, 547–55.

Palisano, R., Rosenbaum, P., Walter, S. et al. (1997). Development and validation of a gross motor function classification system for children with cerebral palsy. *Developmental Medicine and Child Neurology* **39**, 214–23.

Palisano, R., Hanna, S., Rosenbaum, P. et al. (2000). Validation of a model of gross motor function for children with cerebral palsy. *Physical Therapy* **80**, 974–85.

Pless, I.B. and Pinkerton, P. (1975). *Chronic Childhood Disorder. Promoting Patterns of Adjustment*. London: Kimpton.

Robards, M. (1994). *Running a Team for Disabled Children and their Families*. Mac Keith Press. (Distributed by Cambridge University Press.)

Rosenbaum, P. (1988). Children with chronic handicaps: implications for care-giving. In *Redesigning Relationships in Child Health Care, Vol. 2, The Proceedings of a Symposium held February 20–21, 1987*, ed. R.S. Tonkin and J.R. Wright, pp. 134–42. Vancouver: British Columbia Children's Hospital.

Rosenbaum, P.L. (1997). 'Alternative' treatments for children with disabilities: thoughts from the trenches. *Paediatrics and Child Health* **2**, 122–4.

Rosenbaum, P., King, S.M. and Cadman, D. (1992). Measuring processes of caregiving to physically disabled children and families. Part I: identifying relevant components of care. *Developmental Medicine and Child Neurology* **34**, 103–14.

Rosenbaum, P., King, S., Law, M. et al. (1998). Family-centred services: a conceptual framework and research review. *Physical and Occupational Therapy in Pediatrics* **18**, 1–20.

Stewart, D. (1998). *The Transition to Adulthood for Youth with Physical Disabilities: A Qualitative Exploration*. MSc Thesis. Hamilton: McMaster University.

Taylor, D.C. (1982). The components of sickness: diseases, illnesses and predicaments. In *One Child*, ed. J. Apley and C. Ounsted, pp. 1–13. London: Heinemann.

Van Sant, A.F. (1991). Neurodevelopmental treatment and pediatric physical therapy: a commentary. *Pediatric Physical Therapy* **3**, 137–41.

World Health Organization (2001). *International Classification of Impairment, Activity and Participation – ICIDH-2*. Geneva: WHO.

11

Neuropsychological rehabilitation in the community

Pamela Klonoff and David Lamb with further contributions
from Steven Henderson, Lauren Dawson, Jennifer Lutton,
Jessica Grady and Harold Bialsky

Barrow Neurological Institute, Phoenix, Arizona

Introduction

Recovery from brain injury is an extended and arduous process. It is estimated that a full 18 months or more are required to obtain the maximum benefit of natural recovery following a traumatic brain injury (TBI) (Dikmen et al., 1995), while recovering from a stroke can continue for many years (Speach and Dombovy, 1995). Acute rehabilitative efforts for those who have suffered neurological insult typically begin once a patient is judged to be medically stable and transferred to an inpatient rehabilitation unit. Multidisciplinary programmes provide ongoing medical care and seek to address deficits in basic activities of daily living such as orientation, mobility, feeding and communication. Also, an initial assessment of gross cognitive skills is typically conducted. Depending upon progress and perceived need, patients are either discharged home or transferred to a postacute rehabilitation programme. Malec and Basford (1996) provide a hierarchy of the types of brain injury-rehabilitation programmes, with a basic division into subacute and postacute categories. The subacute rehabilitation setting provides long-term residential care for those with such severe deficits that they cannot meaningfully participate in further rehabilitative efforts. These types of people typically include those who require coma management or whose severe behavioural problems preclude ongoing rehabilitation and demand a very intensive level of management.

Malec and Basford (1996) further stratify postacute rehabilitation pro-grammes, with the most restrictive being neurobehavioural programmes. Like subacute management programmes, neurobehavioural programmes work with people who manifest severe behavioural difficulties, but are con-sidered to have the potential to benefit from further rehabilitation. Resi-dential community reintegration programmes are less intensive and focus on vocational goals as well as treating cognitive, emotional, physical and be-havioural deficits. The more intensive outpatient programmes are referred to as comprehensive (holistic) day treatment programmes. These milieu-based neurorehabilitation programmes emphasize the development of a social mi-lieu within the programme and seek to enhance patients' awareness of their residual strengths and brain injury-related difficulties. Outpatient commu-nity re-entry programmes are sometimes also referred to as a Comprehensive Outpatient Rehabilitation Facility (CORF). Such CORF programmes usually house a variety of disciplines in a common location to provide individuali-zed therapeutic services in speech and language pathology, physical therapy, occupational therapy and neuropsychology.

In comparing the available outcome research from these different levels of postacute brain injury-rehabilitation programmes, Malec and Basford (1996) acknowledged the lack of randomized control studies among the research generated in this field. Nonetheless, they concluded there were ben-efits to people who participated in such treatment following brain injury, re-gardless of the type of postacute brain injury-rehabilitation provided. They further noted a better independent work or training outcome in compre-hensive day treatment programmes, ranging between 60% and 80%. By way of comparison, the National Information System tracked the outcomes of 2040 consecutively admitted postacute rehabilitation patients (Evans, 1997). Prior to injury, 93% of this sample were competitive (i.e. employed, attend-ing school or technical training, unsupported homemaker), while only 32% were so classified at discharge.

The following sections will describe a variety of postacute brain injury-rehabilitation approaches in greater detail and provide an overview of the relevant outcome research from each.

Approaches to postacute brain injury rehabilitation

Outpatient community re-entry programmes

CORF programmes emerged approximately 15 to 20 years ago (Malec and Basford, 1996) and were considered postacute services (Evans, 1997). Until that time, patients with traumatic brain injuries were discharged home or to a long-term care institution, and subsequently regressed in their ability to function (Condeluci et al., 1987). There were no services in place to meet the long-term needs of either the disabled person or family members. In 1978, the United States Congress amended the Rehabilitation Act of 1973 to initiate independent living services. This allowed disabled people the opportunity to seek a more meaningful life and enabled rehabilitation therapists the opportunity to provide postacute services.

CORF programmes generally provide selected therapies that focus on circumscribed areas of function. Often people are referred to a CORF pro-gramme after their acute inpatient rehabilitation stay, or alternatively, once they have experienced failures or difficulties with their own attempts at tran-sition to the community (Evans, 1997). They may have reduced stamina and limited awareness of their deficits, and integration into the CORF set-ting allows them to continue their rehabilitation at a pace and level that is commensurate with the acuteness of their injury. The overall goals are to im-prove independent functioning in the home and help with reintegration into the community (e.g. work and/or school). Specific areas addressed include improved mobility, communication and cognitive abilities. The treatment emphasis is on skill application, with the patients learning functional skills in the community and actively compensating for their deficits (Evans, 1997). This would then translate to decreased supervision in the home, improved safety awareness and resumption of pre-injury chores and duties in the home (Evans, 1997). This approach replaced the emphasis on skill reacquisition uti-lized in more acute settings, whereupon the emphasis of treatment was on re-acquiring lost abilities.

Researchers have evaluated the efficacy of the community re-entry app-roach to rehabilitation after traumatic brain injury. Asikainen et al. (1998) studied a group of 508 people referred to an outpatient neurological clinic at Kaunial Hospital in Finland. The mean age was 19 (range 0.8–71 years) and the mean follow-up period was 12 years (range 5 to > 20 years). All of the people admitted to the programme had postinjury problems with education, ability to work or income. Therapy was described as a network of services, including physiotherapy, speech therapy, neuropsychological rehabilitation and occupational therapy. Family members received education and social reintegration before re-employment was attempted. Functional outcome was measured using the Glasgow Outcome Scale (GOS; Jennett and Bond, 1975) and eventual occupational outcome. Results indicated that people with initial mild and moderate brain injuries were capable of working gainfully, as were 70% of those with severe brain injuries between the ages of 17 and 40. Length of coma and duration of posttraumatic amnesia correlated with work history postinjury and with functional outcome measured by the GOS.

Olver et al. (1996) described a sample of 103 people with traumatic brain injuries who completed a comprehensive rehabilitation programme. Patients received both inpatient and outpatient therapies aimed at overcoming disability. Therapies included assistance in obtaining an optimal level of community reintegration that included living situation, vocational productivity and social and recreational activities. At 5 years follow-up, participants had increased their level of independence in use of transportation as well as personal, domestic and community activities of daily living. Specifically, none remained wheelchair-dependent at 5 years. However, 41% of the sample had difficulties with higher-level activities such as running and jumping, and 67% fatigued more easily postinjury with physical exertion. At follow-up, 81% of the sample were performing light domestic chores (e.g. meal preparation, washing dishes, dusting) and 72% were independent with heavy domestic chores (e.g. cleaning, laundry, gardening). Of the sample, 70% were shopping and banking, while 48% were able to drive. More difficulties were encountered with long-term employment, as 32% of those who were employed at 2 years postinjury were not employed at 5 years postinjury. The authors suggested that the employment findings indicate the need for intermittent life-long intervention following traumatic brain injury.

Overall, there is evidence that CORF programmes demonstrate modest to moderate success when they address physical, language and cognitive deficits and actively work with the disabled person and family to improve their level of independence in the home, community and work. What appears to be lacking in this model, however, is the long-term sustenance of employment, suggesting that more intensive treatment approaches are needed to maintain long-term employment (Olver et al., 1996).

Residential and home-based neurorehabilitation

Community-based residential and home-based programmes provide treatment directly in the environment where the person must ultimately reside, presumably producing enhanced clinical outcomes. In general, these programmes address the complex cognitive, social and behavioural problems associated with brain injury while providing appropriate levels of therapeutic support as participants are gradually reintegrated into community and family life. The physical and social environment of these programmes are more likely to be structured in a way that supports the person in the process of learning to perform behaviours and functions necessary for everyday living in one's natural environment (Fryer and Haffey, 1987).

A community-based residential rehabilitation programme typically involves a home-like setting that is generally less costly than traditional inpatient rehabilitation programmes (Cope et al., 1991; Harrick et al., 1994). Harrick and colleagues (1994) describe the Transitional Living Centre of Kingston, Ontario, where people who spent an average of 6 months in the programme demonstrated marked improvements in functional status as indicated by increased productive activity, more independent residential status and decreased level of supervision. These improvements were noted at 1-year follow-up and remained stable or improved at 3-year follow-up. Cope and associates (1991) also reported long-term outcomes for 145 head-injury patients who participated in their postacute rehabilitation programme. These people were found to show significant improvements in residential status, level of productive activity and amount of supervision needed at up to 2 years after discharge. More recently, Gray and Burnham (2000) reported findings from their publicly funded long-term residential rehabilitation programme, the Brain injury rehabilitation programme at Alberta Hospital Ponoka, where participants received an average of 1 year of treatment. Significant improvements were noted, with 85.6% discharged to more independent community living situations.

Eames and colleagues (1995) also found that an average of 11 months treatment in a specialized residential rehabilitation centre was associated with a significant increase in functional independence and a subsequent decrease in long-term costs of care. Johnston and Lewis (1991) reported that the outcomes of a community re-entry programme can be effective in reducing supervision and care requirements for people with traumatic brain injury. Olver (1991) also reported improved domestic and community skills when analysing the outcome of Bethesda Hospital's transitional living centre. In addition, McLaughlin and Peters (1993) found that an innovative transitional phase implemented between inpatient rehabilitation and discharge to the community resulted in more independence in activities of daily living. Willer et al. (1999) reported that people who participated in their residential programme displayed a significant increase in functional abilities following treatment, particularly in motor and cognitive abilities. They also demonstrated greater improvement in community integration. Hedrick and associates (1995) also showed that those in their subacute transitional programme improved after an average of 5 months of treatment. While these outcomes are obviously of benefit to those involved, the fact that these studies focus on increased independence or better functional status instead of gainful employment highlights the typically severe nature of their injuries.

Home-based neurorehabilitation programmes are designed for brain-injured individuals who have achieved medical stability so they can safely pursue their rehabilitation goals at home (Pace et al., 1999). In contrast to traditional home health programmes where people are literally 'homebound', these individuals no longer need to be in the hospital for medical or intensive behavioural treatment, but continue to need varying degrees of coordinated neurorehabilitation services. The intensity of treatment and range of services provided depend on each individual's rehabilitation goals and needs. Services may range from daily rehabilitation services that include physical therapy, occupational therapy, speech therapy and behavioural psychology to weekly services utilizing only one or two of these disciplines. Unlike residential treatment programmes, home-based neurorehabilitation programmes rely on the involvement of family members to provide much of the day-to-day care and implementation of therapies, since they will ultimately be responsible for the patient's long-term care. Home-based programmes also focus on varied services that are tailored to apply to the patient's specific environment, making for better ecological transfer of acquired skills in one's natural setting.

Pace and colleagues (1999) concluded that comprehensive home-based neurorehabilitation appears to be an effective treatment approach, evidenced by the percentage of treatment objectives achieved by people in their programme as well as family and funder satisfaction outcomes with gains maintained at 1-year follow-up. They found that on average, participants met 77% of their objective individual rehabilitation goals at programme discharge. They also found that the percentage of outcomes achieved at 6 months follow-up was 80%, with 78% at 12 months. The authors concluded that these outcomes suggest an enduring benefit of home-based neurorehabilitation.

Community-based residential and home-based rehabilitation programmes are relatively new models of neurorehabilitation that provide an alternative form of treatment for individuals who no longer have medical needs warranting hospitalization but have ongoing cognitive and behavioural remediation needs. Although review of the relevant literature reveals relatively few studies describing community-based residential or home-based rehabilitation programmes and their treatment outcomes, the published studies to date reveal a definite benefit of this type of aftercare for people with brain injuries that provides a positive outcome as well as significant savings in healthcare costs in the long run. In addition, both forms of therapy have been shown to provide benefits that are enduring at limited follow-up intervals.

Supported employment

Supported employment is a type of work placement specifically designed for individuals who, because of their disability, need intensive and ongoing support to perform in a competitive work setting (Gilson, 1998). This form of intervention was initially developed to demonstrate that persons with significant disabilities could be employed competitively if given the proper opportunity and support (Wehman et al., 1995). Although supported employment models were not initially developed for persons with brain injuries, Wehman and Kreutzer (1990) modified the concept of supported employment to meet the needs of brain-injured individuals.

The basic approach of supported employment is to first place the individual in a work setting in order to provide training in the environment in which the work will be performed (Wall et al., 1998). The supported employment model attempts to match the person with a specific job based on their individual attributes, the demands of the position and their own work preferences. Specific interventions include social skills training, job adaptation and modification, counselling, work skills training, and interaction of the rehabilitation professional with the job site. Over time, the rehabilitation professional reduces involvement as the individual improves in independently meeting assigned work duties. 'Extended' services may be required, which include ongoing contacts with the work supervisor and/or specific job skills training or modifications (Wehman et al., 1995). For most people involved in this model of rehabilitation, extended services are available and provided throughout the time they are employed. Other extended services include support services such as psychotherapy, family support, medical services and substance abuse counselling. The advantage of such extended services is that if the job is lost, contact is still ongoing with the vocational services to assist in finding another job (Wehman et al., 1995).

Research by Wehman and associates (1995) evaluated 87 people placed into a supported employment position. They worked an average of 31 hours per week. After programme initiation, there was a steady rate of decline in the percentage of those employed: 78% at 3 months, 59% at 6 months, 53% at 9 months and 51% at 12 months. Other research has found that 38% of a sample was employed 30 months after rehabilitation intervention (Ellerd & Moore, 1992). Wall and colleagues (1998), utilizing a combined work adjustment and supported employment model, studied the outcome of 38 people with brain injury at an average of 18 months after rehabilitation intervention. They found 59% were competitively employed at follow-up. West (1995) found that 19 of 37 people (51%) were employed full-time an average of 6 months after supported employment interventions commenced.

The supported employment model of intervention for persons with brain injury has been praised for its emphasis on self-determination and empowerment while de-emphasizing the pathological models of intervention (Gilson, 1998). Supported employment provides the opportunity for longer provision of services than other more 'traditional' models of vocational intervention, while also enhancing the understanding and acceptance on the part of work settings that extended supports are necessary for patients with brain injury to maintain employment (Goodall and Ghiloni, 2001). The supported employment model appears effective in enabling select patients who have sustained a severe brain injury to return to work.

Milieu-based neurorehabilitation

Comprehensive treatment programmes for persons with brain injury were first developed in Germany after World War I by Walter Poppelreuter and Kurt Goldstein (Uzzell, 2000). As a student of Goldstein in the late 1950s, Yehuda Ben-Yishay combined many of the theories and concepts he learned from Goldstein with his own clinical experiences and thoughts on rehabilitation to create a holistic neurorehabilitation programme for brain-injured Israeli soldiers following the Yom Kippur war in 1973 (Ben-Yishay, 1996). He subsequently developed the Rusk Institute Brain Injury Day Treatment program in New York City, New York, USA (Daniels-Zide and Ben-Yishay, 2000) and allowed other professionals in neurorehabilitation to learn by observing his theories in practice. Among the first to do so was George Prigatano, who took what he learned from Ben-Yishay and created a milieu-based treatment programme first at Presbyterian Hospital in Oklahoma City, Oklahoma, USA (Prigatano et al., 1986) and then at the Barrow Neurological Institute in Phoenix, Arizona, USA (Prigatano et al., 1994). Although limited in number, other milieu-based neurorehabilitation programmes have been established throughout the world. Most of these are described in the recently published *International Handbook of Neuropsychological Rehabilitation* (Christensen and Uzzell, 2000). They include: the centre for Rehabilitation of Brain Injury in Copenhagen, Denmark (Christensen, 2000); the Mayo Medical center Brain Injury Outpatient program in Rochester, Minnesota, USA (Smigielski et al., 1992); the center for Neuropsychological Rehabilitation in Indianapolis, Indiana, USA (Trexler et al., 2000); the Individualized Neuropsychological Subgroup Rehabilitation programme (INSURE) in Helsinki, Finland (Kaipio et al., 2000); the Mulhouse Rehabilitation center of the Delta Group programmes in Mulhouse, France (North et al., 2000); and the Oliver Zangwill centre for Neuropsychological Rehabilitation in Ely, Cambs, UK (Wilson et al., 2000).

The primary tenet of milieu-based neurorehabilitation is that the person's ultimate level of recovery is influenced by the treatment milieu, which is encompassed by the physical, social, and interpersonal environment within which the programme exists (Ben-Yishay, 2000). The personalities, attitudes, and behaviours of the staff, disabled people and support personnel help to create such an environment. As such, admission decisions take into account the makeup of the current milieu and how the individual being considered may potentially impact the milieu. Clinical experience has taught the wisdom of limiting the milieu to no more than two individuals with significant personality disturbances. Also, a mixture of ages seems to be beneficial in that it can enhance cooperation via older people striving to provide a mentoring role to younger brain-injured individuals. Social interaction is encouraged by way of numerous group therapies, hospital-provided lunches 3 days each week, community outings and larger social events such as holiday parties and annual graduation/reunions (Klonoff et al., 2000*a*). A sense of community is also enhanced by group psychotherapy, during which individuals share their feelings about the process of neurorehabilitation and gain a wider perspective when former participants come in to share how their programme experiences affected their ability to function 'in the real world' (Klonoff, 1997).

Many traditional outpatient neurorehabilitation programmes identify themselves as interdisciplinary. However, such programmes would more appropriately be labelled as *multi*disciplinary in that it typically means that services from a variety of disciplines are available within the same facility. In a milieu-based programme, true *inter*disciplinary treatment reflects active collaboration between disciplines. This is achieved by way of five staff meetings each week, during which each person's progress is discussed with input from all disciplines. Moreover, there are certain group therapies that require the involvement of several different disciplines. For example, the vocational counsellor and a speech pathologist run a vocational training group, while a neuropsychologist and speech pathologist conduct an educational group. In addition, for the most part, all disciplines work in cognitive remediation sessions, attend daily milieu sessions and become involved in assisting participants in their work trials. These shared activities provide a foundation of common experiences that allows for better communication and staff cohesion. Finally, staff members are hired based upon their ability to effectively function as part of an interdisciplinary team. This usually requires an open-mindedness to other professional viewpoints, a generally flexible attitude and a willingness to learn about psychological and social dynamics.

Following brain injury, individuals and their families must react to an array of symptoms impacting physical, cognitive, interpersonal and emotional abilities. Such neurological deficits occur within the context of an event that calls into question future goals, including whether the person will be able to return to their former level of educational or vocational functioning (Miller, 1993). Therefore, significant brain injury represents a catastrophic life event not only in the primary effects of the neurologically based deficits, but also in the psychological and interpersonal reactions to the cerebral insult. These secondary problems are typically manifest in greater levels of anxiety, depression and emotional dyscontrol. Premorbid personality characteristics and pre-injury methods of coping will play a critical role in the ability to adapt to these changes (Trexler, 2000). Also, brain injury has an immediate and powerful impact upon the families of people with neurological insult (Curtiss et al., 2000) and the ability of the family to adapt will make a critical contribution to the ultimate outcome (Perlesz et al., 1999). When psychological distress is coupled with the loss of social skills, there is often a gradual increase in social isolation as coworkers, friends and family begin to disengage and avoid extended interactions with the brain-injured person. Both primary and secondary difficulties frequently necessitate radical alterations, which can in turn feed back into the secondary problems. Such a dynamic likely contributes to the finding that caregivers of brain-injured people report a declining quality of life over time (Kolakowsky-Hayner et al., 2001). All of these issues must be addressed if the brain-injured individual is to successfully reintegrate into work and society at large.

Milieu-based neurorehabilitation outcome research

There are a number of examples in the recent literature of research intended to demonstrate improved rehabilitation techniques. For example, using mirrors to provide direct visual feedback was shown to increase functional arm use in a hemiparetic patient (Sathian et al., 2000). Such research efforts are to be lauded for trying to isolate the effects of specific techniques upon recovery from neurological insult. However, individuals rarely present with a single impairment following neurological injury. Most individuals with moderate to severe brain injuries experience multiple neurologically based deficits that exert an influence upon their ability to function, as do the aforementioned secondary psychological and social problems. Therefore, given the necessary multifocal nature of the treatment provided by milieu-based neurorehabilitation programmes, any research focusing on an isolated element of such a programme will fail to address the larger context of the treatment milieu.

Several of the milieu-based rehabilitation programmes have been in existence long enough to provide outcome research. Ben-Yishay et al. (1987) reported an 84% success rate in their ability to return their programme participants to productive activity. At the centre for Rehabilitation of Brain Injury in Copenhagen, Christensen et al. (1992) describe 46 of their early patients; whereby, 70% returned to an education or work setting postdischarge, with the gains being generally maintained at 1-year follow-up. A later study (Christensen, 2000) found that in a sample of 74 people who responded in a follow-up interview 1 to 3 years after discharge, 69% were engaged in work activity. Initial results at the Mayo Medical Center Brain Injury Outpatient Program were also encouraging (Smigielski et al., 1992). Of the 27 people who had completed the programme at that time, 17 (63%) were employed at graduation with one in a permanently supported position, 14 in temporarily supported situations, and two competitively employed. Six of the transitionally employed people had progressed to competitive employment within 1 year of discharge. Research generated at the Adult Day Hospital for Neurological Rehabilitation (ADHNR) is likewise encouraging, and will be described in a separate section below.

Introduction to the ADHNR

In order to illustrate more fully the different elements of milieu-based neurorehabilitation that are considered to contribute to better treatment outcomes, the remainder of this chapter will provide a detailed description of a specific milieu-based programme. The ADHNR has been in operation since January 1986. This form of treatment is modelled after the milieu approach, the conceptual framework of which was derived from the work of Luria (1963, 1974), Ben-Yishay (Ben-Yishay and Prigatano, 1990; Ben-Yishay and Diller, 1993), and Prigatano (Prigatano et al., 1986). There are several basic philosophical goals of the programme that have directed ongoing development of programmatic components as well as current treatment decisions (Klonoff et al., 2000a). The first goal is to improve the individual's level of awareness so that they obtain a thorough understanding of their injury-related strengths and difficulties. The staff then seeks to facilitate acceptance of injury-related changes to assist people in coping with difficulties in functioning. This provides the opportunity to develop realistic, attainable goals, with successful reintegration into their homes, communities and work or school. The success of these rehabilitation efforts is dependent upon the staff's working alliance with the disabled people and their families. A positive working alliance is seen in the capacity of all parties to communicate effectively about overall rehabilitation goals as well as the planning and implementation of appropriate compensatory strategies (Klonoff et al., 2000*b*, 2001).

Description of the ADHNR neurorehabilitation programme

Using the milieu-based approach, individuals participate in a small therapeutic community where they can address the emotional and psychosocial sequelae of their injuries. This is accomplished through extensive small group work at the ADHNR. These group therapies simulate societal demands for cooperation, social appropriateness and accountability in a supportive environment that provides the opportunity to practice integral compensations for productive functioning in the home and community. More specific cognitive, language and physical limitations are addressed in individual therapies.

ADHNR demographics

Since the inception of the ADHNR in 1986, 403 people have participated in the programme. By aetiology, 246 (61.0%) sustained a traumatic brain injury, 52 (12.9%) experienced a stroke, 43 (10.7%) had an aneurysmal or arteriovenous malformation (AVM) rupture, 23 (5.7%) had a brain tumour and 39 (9.7%) had another diagnosis (e.g. anoxia, infection, seizure surgery, etc.). Of those sustaining a TBI, 189 had Glasgow Coma Scale (GCS) scores available in the medical records. Of these, 117 (61.9%) had a GCS of 3–8 (severe), 31 (16.4%) had a GCS of 9–12 (moderate), and 41 (21.7%) had a GCS of 13–15. Thus, the vast majority of people (78.3%) with TBI participating in ADHNR therapies had a moderate to severe TBI.

As for gender, 265 of 403 (66%) participating in ADHNR therapies were men. The average age was 35.5 years (range 14–65), and the average education was 13.7 years (range 2 to over 20). In terms of chronicity (length of time from injury to admission), the average interval was 14.3 months (range = 0.2 to 318), and the median interval was 3.5 months. The length of stay for those participating in therapies was 5.4 months (range = 0.2 to 18.6), and the median length of stay was 4.9 months. A majority of people participated in only one of the available programmes, with 85 (22%) in the Home

Independence programme, 10 (3%) in the School Re-entry programme, and 142 (35%) in the Work Re-entry programme. However, 166 (41%) participated in a combination of these programmes (most typically the Home Independence and Work Re-entry programmes).

Of the 403 who have participated in therapies at the ADHNR, 325 have completed therapies. Thus, 81% of those who began therapies completed an ADHNR therapeutic programme. Reasons for premature discontinuation of treatment include persistent alcohol and/or drug abuse, severe psychiatric problems and poor cooperation/compliance with programme rules and expectations. Of these 325 who completed the programme, 64 (20%) completed the Home Independence programme, 7 (2%) completed the School Re-entry programme, 111 (34%) completed the Work Re-entry programme and 143 (44%) completed a combination of the Home Independence programme and the School and/or Work Re-entry programme. The only significant difference in the data between those completing a programme and those discharged prior to completion was the length of stay, with an average length of stay of 6.2 months for those completing a programme and 2.0 months for those discharged prior to completion.

Overview of the Home Independence programme

The purpose of the Home Independence programme is to help people become as independent as possible at home and in their community (Klonoff et al., 2000a). It is designed for older adolescents and adults who need treatment to improve their independence with self-care tasks and household responsibilities. Many have just been discharged from hospital and initially require 24-hour supervision at home. However, for some it has been months or even years since their injury and they are having difficulties functioning adequately without direct supervision. In either case, they need to learn the appropriate tools and compensations to achieve independence in the home and community. Also, it is critical that the families receive sufficient education and training. Such a clinical observation is congruent with the findings of McPherson et al. (2000), who demonstrated that caregivers of brain-injured people have a strong need for information from neurorehabilitation professionals across a wide variety of topics.

The overall goals of the programme are for participants to conduct daily activities safely and with good judgement both at home and in the community,

Table 11.1. Sample Home Independence checklist

Home Independence Checklist

Due:	Goal:			Achieved:			
Task:	Mon	Tues	Wed	Thurs	Fri	Sat	Sun
1) Make breakfast and clean up daily	___	___	___	___	___	___	___
2) Take medication independently daily	___	___	___	___	___	___	___
3) Do dishes 1×/day	___	___	___	___	___	___	___
4) Clean and dust room 2×/wk	___	___	___	___	___	___	___
5) Vacuum house 1×/wk	___	___	___	___	___	___	___
6) Clean bathroom 1×/wk	___	___	___	___	___	___	___
empty bin							
clean toilet							
wash mirrors							
wash sink							
7) Take out rubbish and recyclables 2×/wk	___	___	___	___	___	___	___
8) Do 3–4 loads laundry/wk	___	___	___	___	___	___	___
9) Check datebook every evening	___	___	___	___	___	___	___
10) Complete home exercises 3–4×/wk	___	___	___	___	___	___	___
11) Write in journal every evening	___	___	___	___	___	___	___
12) Complete weekly meal plan 1×/wk	___	___	___	___	___	___	___
13) Help with the grocery shopping 1×/wk	___	___	___	___	___	___	___
14) Prepare simple meal independently 1×/wk	___	___	___	___	___	___	___

Patient's signature	Family member's signature

to become as productive as possible at home while remaining unsupervised for at least 4 hours, and to learn appropriate compensations to help achieve independence (Klonoff et al., 2000*a*). To address these goals and monitor progress, home visits, community outings and a Home Independence checklist are utilized (see Table 11.1).

The Home Independence checklist is utilized with almost every person in the Home Independence programme (Klonoff et al., 2000*a*). It is a compensatory strategy intended to help people organize their day, recall specific details necessary for completion of each job, stay focused upon the task at hand, and become independent with daily self-care and household management tasks. The checklist is developed with both the disabled person and family, keeping in mind previous domestic responsibilities as well as their current level of functioning. It usually begins with only a few tasks and gradually increases in the number and complexity of tasks. The checklist is utilized to help the person become as independent as possible, with the goal

Table 11.2. Procedural checklist for paying bills

Bill Paying Checklist

Step	Date					
1) Tear off portion of bill to mail						
2) Fill in blanks on bill about amount to be paid						
3) Write date on cheque						
4) Write name in "Pay to the order of" on cheque						
5) Write amount on cheque						
6) Sign cheque						
7) Write bill account # and name in cheque memo						
8) Write payment info on our portion of the bill						
9) Write check info in cheque register before putting cheque in envelope						
10) Put cheque and payment stub in envelope						
11) Put postage on envelope						
12) Put our portion of the bill in box to file						
13) Put bill in bank bag or datebook to be mailed						

of resuming all or most of their previous responsibilities. It also provides the necessary structure to achieve a successful daily routine.

Another important compensation that is used with everyone in the Home Independence programme is the datebook. The datebook is utilized as a memory compensation to help organize the daily schedule, keep track of appointments and important information and record how they spend their day. After the initial evaluation, an appropriate datebook is recommended according to the severity of memory difficulties and anticipated level of responsibility. They are trained on how to utilize the datebook effectively, learning a variety of helpful strategies and techniques (Kime et al., 1996). They are also given numerous memory assignments to practice their skills and to see where they are having difficulty.

Other compensations may also be utilized, depending on the nature of their responsibilities as well as their level of functioning. These may include a weekly meal plan, categorized grocery list, cash tracking sheet and other money management compensations. More specific checklists are often created for subroutines such as doing the laundry, printing out schedules from the computer or paying bills (see Table 11.2). After the compensations are set in place, the next step is to integrate them into the home and community.

This involves regular home visits and a variety of community outings. The home visits involve developing the Home Independence checklist, making modifications to compensations as needed, observing utilization of the compensations, organizational tasks such as setting up a filing system, and family education and training.

Overview of the Work Re-Entry programme

Work re-entry begins early in the rehabilitation process and can be found in any number of elements within the ADHNR treatment milieu (Klonoff et al., 2000a). An initial 2-week multidisciplinary assessment provides clues about a person's potential to return to work. However, understanding of such testing data must be tempered by other factors, such as acuteness of injury, whether the person is trying to return to a former position or find an entirely new job, the exact nature of their anticipated job responsibilities and their and their family's attitudes toward returning to work.

Answers to the questions of how these factors impact work re-entry can be found in a variety of therapies. Cognitive Retraining is a series of novel tasks that are presented during the first session of the treatment day (Klonoff et al., 1989, 1997). Since most of these tasks are carefully measured, it is possible to estimate relative speed of thinking, attention to detail, proneness to errors and reaction time (Klonoff et al., 1989). By observing the way in which people approach learning these activities, valuable information is gathered relative to their ability to use compensations, level of distractibility, procedural memory, social appropriateness and other critical areas of functioning not usually assessed during formal testing (Klonoff et al., 1989, 1997). Through lecture-style presentations and subsequent quizzes given in Cognitive Group, staff members are able to evaluate the ability to learn new information, which obviously has implications for the return to school, but also may be important in rapidly evolving fields (e.g. information technology) or careers requiring rapid acquisition of new knowledge (e.g. attorneys). Communication skills and social pragmatics are dealt with in a variety of other groups, including Vocational/Communication Group, Current Events, Datebook Group, Milieu, and Group Psychotherapy. Physical readiness to work is addressed during group and individual Physical and Occupational Therapy sessions. Finally, emotional readiness is assessed via exploration of feelings about the job and awareness of the functional impact of their deficit areas in Individual and Group Psychotherapy (Klonoff, 1997).

Once a person is considered ready for work, the vocational counsellor becomes actively involved in the treatment. If a new position is to be found, job development is the primary focus, with staff helping to narrow the focus to the types of jobs consistent with postinjury skills, interests and deficits. Work re-entry also involves returning people to their former place of employment whenever possible. This usually begins with a meeting between treatment staff and representatives from the workplace.

Once the person has begun working, hours at the job gradually increase while the schedule at the ADHNR decreases. There is a heavy on-site presence by treatment staff early in the work trial process (generally for the first 6 to 12 weeks), to help with developing specific compensations and providing support during what is frequently an anxiety-provoking situation. If necessary, the staff help to develop modifications in job duties and/or position descriptions so as to accommodate postinjury abilities. Even after a person has successfully returned to a full-time work schedule, the programme makes weekly contact with the direct supervisor for the next 1 to 2 months to ensure everyone is satisfied regarding level of job performance before effecting formal discharge from the ADHNR. Often intermittent contact with the employer continues for an extended period after formal discharge and is available as long as is necessary.

Overview of ADHNR research

Previous work by Klonoff et al. (2000*b*) examined the role of milieu-based interdisciplinary neurorehabilitation on vocational outcome at up to 11 years postdischarge in 112 people who had sustained moderate to severe traumatic brain injuries. Using a cross-sectional design, 'productivity' and 'competitive activity' were measured at follow-up intervals of 3 months and 1, 3, 5, 7, 9 and 11 years. 'Productivity' was defined as gainful employment, school and/or volunteer work, with 'competitive activity' being defined as work for pay or enrolment in school.

Former participants were contacted by telephone by an objective rater at each of the aforementioned follow-up intervals. When contacted at multiple follow-up data points, outcome data for the time furthest from discharge were used in the analyses. As a result, independent samples were used at each follow-up period. People were classified into one of ten categories at follow-up: (1) full-time work, (2) full-time school, (3) full-time work and school, (4) part-time work, (5) part-time school, (6) full-time volunteer, (7) part-time volunteer, (8) homemaker, (9) retired and (10) not working. Of note, the homemaker category was considered productive because of the complexity and demands of managing a household. The retired category was considered nonproductive because most of these people were forced into retirement as a consequence of their brain injury.

Analyses revealed that 88.4% of the participants in this study were productive postdischarge, and 76.8% of these persons were engaged in competitive activity. Another encouraging result from this study was the finding that there was no decline in the level of either productive or competitive activity as a function of elapsed time during the 11-year follow-up period. Klonoff and her colleagues (2000b) attributed their findings to a number of treatment variables that included the programme's milieu-based components emphasizing increased awareness of injury-related difficulties and facilitation of socially appropriate behaviours as well as the use of individual and group psychotherapy sessions to help people accept alternative career goals. They also acknowledged the role of the work environment in facilitating a positive outcome, with better outcomes being achieved in more flexible work settings that allow the use of compensations in the work place.

More recently, Klonoff et al. (2001) expanded their former study to examine the effects of milieu-based neurorehabilitation in a larger population with heterogeneous brain injuries. In addition to the aforementioned traumatic brain-injury sample, people suffering from cerebrovascular accidents, brain resection secondary to brain tumour or intractable epilepsy, encephalitis and anoxia were also included in the study. The former analyses were also expanded to investigate additional variables of interest, such as the impact on vocational outcome of process variables like the working alliance ratings between participants and staff members. Using the same research design described above, individuals were contacted by telephone by an objective rater to collect postdischarge data at 3 months and 1, 3, 5, 7, 9 and 11 years. A total of 164 people were included in this study and similar groupings of productivity and competitive activity were determined.

Data analyses revealed that 83.5% of those in this study were productive postdischarge, with 67.1% of the sample involved in some form of gainful work or school. Again, no decline in level of productive activity was evident as a function of the time elapsed since discharge. In reference to process variables of interest, higher staff ratings of working alliance with participants and their families were associated with an increased level of long-term productivity and improved work status. Younger age, but not level of education, was also found to relate to improved levels of long-term productivity.

Overall, both of these studies suggest that a large majority of people undergoing a comprehensive milieu-based neurorehabilitation programme are productive in some gainful capacity up to 11 years postdischarge with no significant decline in functioning over this time period. Such an outcome argues for the enduring benefits of milieu-oriented rehabilitation.

Summary

This chapter has reviewed various models of postacute rehabilitation for individuals with brain injury. Treatment approaches reviewed include CORF, community-based residential and home-based rehabilitation, supported employment and milieu-based rehabilitation. The characteristics of each approach were reviewed as well as some of the relevant outcome data.

Based on our clinical experience and review of the literature, each approach has some benefit to a particular subgroup of the brain-injured population. Individuals with milder injuries and more circumscribed deficits appear to benefit from a CORF programme. Those with very severe brain injuries who may otherwise be institutionalized benefit from a community-based residential or home-based neurorehabilitation programme. The supported employment model is most applicable to persons who need ongoing external support in order to maintain long-term employment.

The milieu-based neurorehabilitation programme provides a comprehensive, holistic approach that is particularly effective in addressing cognitive, behavioural, interpersonal and psychosocial sequelae of brain injury. The milieu-based neurorehabilitation programme has been effective in maintaining high levels of gainful employment and productivity even at 11 years postdischarge (Klonoff et al., 2001). The success of this approach can be attributed to its holistic orientation that incorporates multiple aspects embedded in the other treatment models described above, including independent functioning in the home and community utilizing home visits and ongoing therapeutic supervision in the workplace.

Acknowledgements

We would like to thank Marley Kornreich for her invaluable assistance with data transcription and data entry.

REFERENCES

Asikainen, I., Kaste, M. and Sarna, S. (1998). Predicting late outcome for patients with traumatic brain injury referred to a rehabilitation programme: a study of 508 Finnish patients 5 years or more after injury. *Brain Injury* **12**, 95–107.

Ben-Yishay, Y. (1996). Reflections on the evolution of the therapeutic milieu concept. *Neuropsychological Rehabilitation* **6**, 327–43.

Ben-Yishay, Y. (2000). Postacute neuropsychological rehabilitation: a holistic perspective. In *International Handbook of Neuropsychological Rehabilitation*, ed. A-L. Christensen and B.P. Uzzell, pp. 127–35. New York: Plenum Publishers.

Ben-Yishay, Y. and Diller, L. (1993). Cognitive remediation in traumatic brain injury: update and issues. *Archives of Physical Medicine and Rehabilitation* **74**, 204–13.

Ben-Yishay, Y. and Prigatano, G.P. (1990). Cognitive remediation. In *Rehabilitation of the Adult and Child with Traumatic Brain Injury*, ed. M. Rosenthal, E.R. Griffith, M.R. Bond and J.D. Miller, 2nd edn, pp. 393–409. Philadelphia: F.A. Davis.

Ben-Yishay, Y., Silver, S.M., Piasetsky, E. and Rattock, J. (1987). Relationship between employability and vocational outcome after intensive holistic cognitive rehabilitation. *Journal of Head Trauma Rehabilitation* **24**, 33–43.

Christensen, A-L. (2000). Neuropsychological postacute rehabilitation. In *International Handbook of Neuropsychological Rehabilitation*, ed. A-L. Christensen and B.P. Uzzell, pp. 151–63. New York: Plenum Publishers.

Christensen, A-L., Pinner, E.M., Pedersen, P.M., Teasdale, T.W. and Trexler, L.E. (1992). Psychosocial outcome following individualized neuropsychological rehabilitation of brain damage. *Acta Neurologica Scandinavica* **85**, 32–8.

Christensen, A-L. and Uzzell, B.P. (2000). *International Handbook of Neuropsychological Rehabilitation*. New York: Plenum Publishers.

Condeluci, A., Cooperman, S. and Seif, B.A. (1987). Independent living: settings and supports. In *Community Re-entry for Head Injured Adults*, ed. M. Ylvisaker and E.M.R. Gobble, pp. 301–47. Boston, MA: College-Hill Press.

Cope, D.N., Cole, J.R., Hall, K.M. and Barkin, H. (1991). Brain injury: analysis of outcome in a post-acute rehabilitation system, Part I: General analysis. *Brain Injury* **5**, 111–25.

Curtiss, G., Klemz, S. and Vanderploeg, R.D. (2000). Acute impact of severe traumatic brain injury on family structure and coping responses. *Journal of Head Trauma Rehabilitation* **15**, 1113–22.

Daniels-Zide, E. and Ben-Yishay, Y. (2000). Therapeutic milieu day programme. In *International Handbook of Neuropsychological Rehabilitation*, ed. A-L. Christensen and B.P. Uzzell, pp. 183–93. New York: Plenum Publishers.

Dikmen, S.S., Machamer, J.E., Winn, H.R. and Temkin, N.R. (1995). Neuropsychological outcome at 1-year post head injury. *Neuropsychology* **9**, 80–90.

Eames, P., Cotterill, G., Kneale, T.A., Storrar, A.L. and Yeomans, P. (1995). Outcome of intensive rehabilitation after severe brain injury: a long term follow-up study. *Brain Injury* **10**, 631–50.

Ellerd, D.A. and Moore, S.C. (1992). Follow-up at twelve and thirty months of persons with traumatic brain injury engaged in supported employment placements. *Journal of Applied Rehabilitation Counseling* **23**, 48–50.

Evans, R.W. (1997). Postacute neurorehabilitation: roles and responsibilities within a national information system. *Archives of Physical Medicine and Rehabilitation* **78** (Suppl. 4), S17–25.

Fryer, L.J. and Haffey, W.J. (1987). Cognitive rehabilitation and community readaptation: outcomes from two program models. *Journal of Head Trauma Rehabilitation* **2**, 51–63.

Gilson, S.F. (1998). Case management and supported employment: a good fit. *Journal of Case Management* **7**, 10–17.

Goodall, P. and Ghiloni, C.T. (2001). The changing face of publicly funded employment services. *Journal of Head Trauma Rehabilitation* **16**, 94–106.

Gray, D.S. and Burnham, R.S. (2000). Preliminary outcomes analysis of a long-term rehabilitation program for severe acquired brain injury. *Archives of Physical Medicine and Rehabilitation* **81**, 1447–56.

Harrick, L., Krefting, L., Johnston, J., Carlson, P. and Minnes, P. (1994). Stability and functional outcomes following transitional living programme participation: 3-year follow-up. *Brain Injury* **8**, 439–47.

Hedrick, W.P., Pickleman, H.L. and Walker, W. (1995). Analysis of demographic and functional subacute (transitional) rehabilitation data. *Brain Injury* **9**, 563–73.

Jennett, B. and Bond, M. (1975). Assessment of outcome after severe brain injury damage. *Lancet* **1**, 480–7.

Johnston, M.V. and Lewis, F.D. (1991). Outcomes of community re-entry programs for brain injury survivors, Part 1: Independent living and productive activities. *Brain Injury* **5**, 141–54.

Kaipio, M-L., Sarajuuri, J. and Koskinen, S. (2000). The INSURE program and modifications in Finland. In *International Handbook of Neuropsychological Rehabilitation*, ed. A-L. Christensen and B.P. Uzzell, pp. 247–58. New York: Plenum Publishers.

Kime, S.K., Lamb, D.G. and Wilson, B.A. (1996). Use of a comprehensive programme of external cueing to enhance procedural memory in a patient with dense amnesia. *Brain Injury* **10**, 17–25.

Klonoff, P.S. (1997). Individual and group psychotherapy in milieu oriented rehabilitation. *Applied Neuropsychology* **4**, 107–18.

Klonoff, P.S., O'Brien, K.P., Chiapello, D.A, Prigatano, G.P. and Cunningham, M. (1989). Cognitive retraining after traumatic brain injury and its role in facilitating awareness. *Journal of Head Trauma Rehabilitation* **4**, 37–45.

Klonoff, P.S., Lamb, D.G., Chiapello, D.A. et al. (1997). Cognitive retraining in a milieu-oriented program. In *Theoretical Foundations of Clinical Neuropsychology for Clinical Practitioners*, ed. M.E. Maruish and J.A. Moses, pp. 219–36. Mahwah, NJ: Lawrence Erlbaum.

Klonoff, P.S., Lamb, D.G., Henderson, S.W., Reichert, M.V. and Tully, S.L. (2000*a*). Milieu-based neurorehabilitation at the Adult Day Hospital for Neurological Rehabilitation. In *International Handbook of Neuropsychological Rehabilitation*, ed. A-L. Christensen and B.P. Uzzell, pp. 195–213. New York: Plenum Publishers.

Klonoff, P.S., Lamb, D.G. and Henderson, S.W. (2000*b*). Outcome from milieu-based neurorehabilitation in patients with traumatic brain injury at up to eleven years post-discharge. *Archives of Physical Medicine and Rehabilitation* **81**, 1535–7.

Klonoff, P.S., Lamb, D.G. and Henderson, S.W. (2001). Outcomes from milieu-based rehabilitation at up to 11 years post-discharge. *Brain Injury* **15**, 413–28.

Kolakowsky-Hayner, S.A., Miner, K.D. and Kreutzer, J.S. (2001). Long-term life quality and family needs after traumatic brain injury. *Journal of Head Trauma Rehabilitation* **16**, 374–85.

Luria, R.A. (1963). *Restoration of Function after Brain Injury*. New York: MacMillan.

Luria, R.A. (1974). *The Working Brain*. London: Penguin Press.

Malec, J.F. and Basford, J.S. (1996). Postacute brain injury-rehabilitation. *Archives of Physical Medicine and Rehabilitation* **77**, 198–207.

McLaughlin, A.M. and Peters, S. (1993). Evaluation of an innovative cost-effective program for brain injury patients: response to need for flexible treatment planning. *Brain Injury* **7**, 71–5.

McPherson, K.M., McNaughton, H. and Pentland, B. (2000). Information needs of families when one member has a severe brain injury. *International Journal of Rehabilitation Research* **23**, 295–301.

Miller, L. (1993). *Psychotherapy of the Brain-injured Patient: Reclaiming the Shattered Self.* New York: W.W. Norton.

North, P., Passadori, A. and Millemann, P. (2000). The Delta Group experience: TBI in France. In *International Handbook of Neuropsychological Rehabilitation*, ed. A-L. Christensen and B.P. Uzzell, pp. 273–81. New York: Plenum Publishers.

Olver, J. (1991). Towards community re-entry. *Think* **1**, 28–9.

Olver, J.H., Ponsford, J.L. and Curran, C.A. (1996). Outcome following traumatic brain injury: A comparison between 2 and 5 years after injury. *Brain Injury* **10**, 841–8.

Pace, G.M., Schlund, M.W., Hazard-Haupt, T. et al. (1999). Characteristics and outcomes of a home and community-based neurorehabilitation programme. *Brain Injury* **13**, 535–46.

Perlesz, A., Kinsella, G. and Crowe, S. (1999). Impact of traumatic brain injury on the family: a critical review. *Rehabilitation Psychology* **44**, 6–35.

Prigatano, G.P., Fordyce, D.J., Zeiner, H.K. et al. (1986). *Neuropsychological Rehabilitation after Traumatic Brain Injury*. Baltimore: Johns Hopkins University Press.

Prigatano, G.P., Klonoff, P.S., O'Brien, K.P. et al. (1994). Productivity after neuropsychologically oriented milieu rehabilitation. *Journal of Head Trauma Rehabilitation* **9**, 91–102.

Sathian, K., Greenspan, A.I. and Wolf, S.L. (2000). Doing it with mirrors: a case study of a novel approach to neurorehabilitation. *Neurorehabilitation and Neural Repair* **14**, 73–6.

Smigielski, J.S., Malec, J.F., Thompson, J.M. and DePompolo, R.W. (1992). Mayo Medical Center Brain Injury Outpatient program: treatment procedures and early outcome data. *Mayo Clinical Process* **67**, 767–74.

Speach, D.P. and Dombovy, M.L. (1995). Recovery from stroke: rehabilitation. *Baillieres Clinical Neurology* **4**, 317–38.

Trexler, L.E. (2000). Empirical support for neuropsychological rehabilitation. In *International Handbook of Neuropsychological Rehabilitation*, ed. A-L. Christensen and B.P. Uzzell, pp. 137–50. New York: Plenum Publishers.

Trexler, L.E., Eberle, R. and Zappalá, G. (2000). Models and programs of the Center for Neuropsychological Rehabilitation: fifteen years experience. In *International Handbook of Neuropsychological Rehabilitation*, ed. A-L. Christensen and B.P. Uzzell, pp. 215–29. New York: Plenum Publishers.

Uzzell, B.P. (2000). Neuropsychological rehabilitation. In *International Handbook of Neuropsychological Rehabilitation*, ed. A-L. Christensen and B.P. Uzzell, pp. 353–69. New York: Plenum Publishers.

Wall, J.R, Rosenthal, M. and Niemczura, J.G. (1998). Community-based training after acquired brain injury: preliminary findings. *Brain Injury* **12**, 215–24.

Wehman, P. and Kreutzer, J.S. (1990). *Vocational Rehabilitation for Persons with Traumatic Brain Injury*. Rockville, MD: Aspen Publishers.

Wehman, P.H., West, M.D., Kregel, J., Sherron, P. and Kreutzer, J.S. (1995). Return to work for persons with severe traumatic brain injury: a data-based approach to program development. *Journal of Head Trauma and Rehabilitation* **10**, 27–39.

West, M.D. (1995). Aspects of workplace and return to work for persons with brain injury in supported employment. *Brain Injury* **9**, 301–13.

Willer, B., Button, J. and Rempel, R. (1999). Residential and home-based postacute rehabilitation of individuals with traumatic brain injury: a case control study. *Archives of Physical Medicine and Rehabilitation* **80**, 399–406.

Wilson, B.A., Evans, J., Brentnall, S. et al. (2000). The Oliver Zangwill Center for Neuropsychological Rehabilitation: a partnership between health care and rehabilitation research. In *International Handbook of Neuropsychological Rehabilitation*, ed. A-L. Christensen and B.P. Uzzell, pp. 231–46. New York: Plenum Publishers.

12

The way forward

The aim of this chapter is to pull together the various strands of the book and point to a way forward for future service development and research.

The aim of this book has been to make the case for increasing resources, services and facilities to be placed in a community setting for the benefit of disabled people. We hope that the theoretical case has been made throughout the chapters in this book. However, we also hope that a partial academic case has been made by a comprehensive review of the community neurological rehabilitation research literature. This review has made it clear to us, and probably to the reader, that much more work needs to be done in this field. There is a paucity of adequate studies of the different models of service delivery. Many theoretical models have never been subject to any rigorous evaluation. This is not to suggest that there is a single model of community rehabilitation as this is certainly not the case. Each individual community may have a number of appropriate models that could be developed depending on their own resources, existing hospital facilities, existing community networks as well as their own sense of local community and local culture.

Such literature that has been reviewed has largely had a health focus. There is even less evaluation of broader-based social models of independent living. There are plenty of theories and opinions about the way disabled people should interact with health and social professionals but there is a dearth of research knowledge, either quantitative or qualitative, as to how this interaction can best be taken forward. Many questions remain to be answered. Exactly how can disabled people be effectively involved in service planning? How can the views of disabled people be most effectively incorporated into the rehabilitation goal-setting process? How do we best deal with conflicts that arise between the health professionals themselves and more particularly between the disabled person and the rehabilitation team? How can we improve the knowledge base of disabled people and what is the most effective way of information sharing? Which particular model of service delivery is the most efficacious for a particular type of disability? How can a rehabilitation team best support carers and/or the children of disabled people? These are just some of the key questions that need addressing and answering in the coming years so that our knowledge of community rehabilitation can be advanced for the benefit of all concerned.

We are particularly conscious that many mistakes in the development of community services have been made, albeit in a different context, in the South. We strongly believe that many lessons can be learnt from the successes, and from the mistakes, in these CBR programmes. The clear, and obvious, message is that any community rehabilitation programme should actively seek the participation of disabled people and preferably such programmes should be designed by, and supervised by, local disabled people. However, it is just as important for the whole community to be involved in the project as much as possible. This may mean that community rehabilitation is delivered in, for example, a local community centre or that information and educational groups meet in the local library. It is only by such means that inappropriate, or even hostile, societal attitudes can slowly be broken down. The other particular lesson to be learnt from Southern CBR projects is with regard to professional flexibility and the avoidance of strict professional boundaries. As rehabilitation moves into the community then professional boundaries have to become more indistinct. The compartmentalization of professional interests has some relevance in an acute setting but not in a community setting. For example, a physiotherapist seeing someone at home clearly needs to be aware of broader, nonphysiotherapy issues. It would be counter to the underlying philosophy of community rehabilitation if the physiotherapist simply concentrated on transfers or stair climbing when the disabled person wished to discuss kitchen adaptations or wanted the address of the local Stroke Club. The physiotherapist may not have such information but undoubtedly needs to be part of a team that does have such expertise. Thus, this book has pointed towards the concept of the generic therapist. While such an individual may have a particular professional qualification their professional role needs to be much broader.

We believe the evidence points to the case for such broad-based training in community rehabilitation – perhaps as a postgraduate qualification. At the same time we are aware that while professionals clearly have a major role in the community rehabilitation team, many of the day-to-day rehabilitation goals can be delivered through rehabilitation assistants and by properly trained and informed members of the family and, as appropriate, disabled people themselves. Thus, the literature points not only to the development of a broad-based qualified professional but also to a broad-based generic rehabilitation assistant. Such roles clearly require high-quality training and maintenance of standards, which currently do not exist.

Another clear conclusion from review of the literature is the unnecessary organizational boundaries that exist between health and social services. In some countries, such as Northern Ireland, such boundaries do not exist and while we accept that there is no evidence that managerial merger of these services produces a better service, common sense dictates that this must be the case. However, we are aware that common sense does not amount to strong evidence and certainly research needs to be encouraged to compare outcomes, quantitatively and qualitatively, where such organizational boundaries have been blurred or broken down. Nevertheless, it is also clear that other relevant government departments need to be integrated within the long-term rehabilitation support network. This is particularly true for employment but can also apply to the educational sector, housing sector and indeed the charitable and voluntary agencies. Once again there is a dearth of literature on fully integrated service models. Examples exist, as described in Chapters 7 and 9, of effective working practices but it is clear that there is little cross-fertilization of ideas, let alone staff and budgets, between the different experts and the different government and private agencies.

Illustrative case histories – what might have happened

In Chapter 1 the authors gave four illustrative case histories from their local experience. In all these cases there were considerable problems caused by lack of appropriate community rehabilitation. It is interesting to speculate what the outcome might have been had appropriate community support been in place.

Case study 1

> Mr B was a 67-year-old retired railway worker who looked after his mildly disabled wife. He had no family but a good local network of neighbours. He had a stroke causing profound left hemiparesis and visual and sensory neglect requiring his acute admission to hospital. After a couple of weeks in hospital he had become depressed and developed a pressure sore, which then became infected with methicillin-resistant *staphylococcus aureus* (MRSA). After around 2 months he was eventually referred to the rehabilitation centre where he had a rather long and slow rehabilitation, which was hampered by his need to remain on a pressure-relieving mattress and further complicated by his need to be nursed in his own room because of the MRSA infection. He eventually had a good outcome and was discharged back home to continue looking after his wife, around 6 months after his stroke.

The problem in this case occurred after 2 weeks in the acute hospital. At that point the limited therapy that had been available on the acute ward was beginning to be withdrawn as the sole physiotherapist had to spend more time with more acutely ill patients. At the same time Mr B was becoming depressed, probably by a combination of his stroke and concern over his wife who needed support from neighbours. Mr B seems an ideal case for support by an early discharge team. If he had been discharged to the care of such a team around 2 weeks after his stroke his pressure sore may well have been prevented. It seems likely that his depression and his general reluctance to participate in any active rehabilitation led to more prolonged periods in bed and, on a busy acute ward, led to the development of the pressure sore. An early-discharge stroke team should have been able to deliver ongoing physiotherapy in his home environment. Mr B would presumably have been less anxious as he was at home with his wife. If he was not able to look after her as usual then the stroke team should have been able to organize some social care and home help for the couple. The stroke team should include a neuropsychologist who may have been able to provide some more detailed assessment of Mr B's disability and perhaps the complicating features of the sensory and visual neglect would have been recognized and explained. The incipient depression may have been picked up earlier and appropriate interventions arranged. Thus, with luck, by these means the complication of his pressure sore and significant delay in his rehabilitation would have been prevented. Mr B would have been more at ease at home with his wife and there would have been less stress both on his wife and also on the neighbours who had to rally round for 6 months to look after her.

Case study 2

Mrs W was a 78-year-old teacher who had a mild stroke resulting in a right hemiparesis and dysarthria. She was felt not to be disabled enough to be admitted to an acute hospital and indeed being an independent-minded lady was reluctant to move from her home. Regrettably spasticity slowly worsened her gait and she became more housebound. In addition she was embarrassed about her dysarthria and disliked communicating with friends or shopkeepers. The situation had slowly worsened and she developed incontinence as a result of her difficulties getting around the house. Finally, the situation was complicated by depression causing her to be admitted to the local nursing home.

How could this situation have been prevented? It seems in this case that Mrs W was an ideal candidate for support by a community-based team. A resource team for the elderly may have been able to give her the necessary social support and provide home help such that shopping and housework could have been done without the need to call on her neighbours. The physiotherapist on the team should have been able to monitor the development of spasticity and prevent deterioration in her gait and thus indirectly prevent the onset of incontinence. It may simply have been that such physiotherapy and social support would have prevented the onset of depression but even if this had been a complicating factor then the necessary social and counselling support from a resource team may have been able to provide appropriate antidepressant intervention. Good-quality rehabilitation may also have provided some assistance for her embarrassing dysarthria. If the resource team was able to have access to both health and social service budgets then the combined rehabilitation support and social support could have been put in place swiftly and quickly and it seems likely that Mrs W would have been able to live in her own home for much longer than was the actual case.

Case study 3

Mrs M was a 33-year-old lady with multiple sclerosis. She had remained reasonably well until the previous 2 years when she had had three relapses each of which required admission to hospital. She had made a reasonably good recovery from the relapses although she was left with a mild degree of spastic paraparesis, bladder difficulties and very early ataxia of her hands and speech. She lived at home with her two young girls and her husband worked away on the oil rigs. She was admitted to hospital for her relapses, which regrettably caused some family problems as her girls needed looking after by Mrs M's sister and her repeated absence from work caused her considerable problems when her employer dismissed her. She is now also involved in an industrial tribunal claim for unfair dismissal.

This is the sort of complex and unsatisfactory situation that can arise when individuals with ongoing neurological disabilities have no long-term rehabilitation support. Mrs M only had support from the acute neurology service and to access their assistance she required to be admitted to hospital. If there had been a local community multiple sclerosis team then perhaps these difficulties may not have arisen. The team should have had physiotherapy input to assist with her relapse and may well have had access to a rehabilitation physician or MS nurse who could have administered the intravenous steroids within her home environment. It should have been possible for the steroids to be administered outside work hours and she may not have needed time off work. A home support worker may have assisted in looking after her children and undertaking some of the household jobs while Mrs M was less able to do so. This would have prevented additional family strain as the need for her sister to look after her children while she was in hospital would not have arisen. This is also a situation where liaison with the employer may have been helpful. A relevant member of the MS team may have been able to talk to the employer and explain the nature of her condition. It may well have been that she would have remained a good employee for many years to come if the employer understood the nature of the condition and thus been able to be a little more flexible with regard to occasional days off work or occasional periods of part-time working over acute relapses. A useful employee may have been retained and further strain on Mrs M would have been avoided as she would hopefully have not ended up with the trauma of an industrial tribunal.

Case study 4

This case study illustrated an unfortunately common result of brain injury. Often there is good physical recovery after such injuries but individuals have very significant difficulties as a result of behavioural, cognitive and intellectual problems. Mr Y had severe behavioural disturbance in the early weeks after his injury complicated by significant difficulties with short-term memory, poor concentration, slowed information-processing speed, disorganization and the need for constant prompting, guidance and supervision. He was initially in a safe and appropriate environment in a regional brain-injury centre. It is likely that if he had been persuaded to stay in the centre an active behavioural re-habilitation programme would have produced eventual benefit. However, time was not available as Mr Y discharged himself from the unit with the active support of his parents. It was not felt that Mr Y could be kept against his will in the unit as while he was ag-gressive he was not a significant danger to himself or others. However, the situation was clearly fraught and the home situation broke down and Mr Y moved in with his girlfriend and small child. This situation did not last either and Mr Y moved into a hostel and into the world of crime. He was fortunate not to receive a custodial sentence for stealing a car and eventually moved out of the area.

It is quite likely that this situation could have been prevented by ongo-ing community support. A community-based head-injury team may well have been able to provide an outpatient behavioural programme within the home environment. It may well have been that in this environment, with the assistance of his parents, the regime would have been more successful. Mr Y may have felt more comfortable and at ease in his home surroundings and perhaps the parents and his girlfriend could have been persuaded to participate in the behavioural programme. A neuropsychologist could have organized an appropriate regime and it is quite possible that one of the other team members could have worked actively with Mr Y in terms of his day-to-day requirements for prompting, guidance and general supervision. It is likely that if such input could have been carried on for a few months in the home then Mr Y would have recovered sufficiently either to remain at home or to move more successfully in with his girlfriend and her small child. The parents and his girlfriend may have received counselling support and an explanation of the problems, which might have enabled them to deal with the difficulties more effectively. He might have been prevented from drifting into a life of crime. Even if this had not been possible then better liaison with the police might have prevented his case from going to court. Ongoing vocational rehabilitation may have enabled Mr Y to take advantage of local employment opportunities from sympathetic employers.

These cases studies illustrate some of the real difficulties that can arise without appropriate community rehabilitation. While the cases are based on real experiences the suggested solutions are fictitious. Nevertheless these studies illustrate the clear value that may follow from appropriate rehabilitation delivered in a community setting.

We are aware that this book has probably produced more questions than answers. We hope it has stimulated interest in the subject and encouraged others to become involved in the field either clinically or from an educational or research perspective. We hope some of these questions will have been answered in a few years' time, and we can put them in a second edition of the book! We hope by then that community neurological rehabilitation will be an accepted part of neurological and rehabilitation practice. We hope it will have become fully integrated, not only with acute hospital rehabilitation units, but also with a whole range of other community professionals and, most particularly, integrated with disabled people's groups. Many changes will need to wait for legislative reorganization but goodwill and cooperation between interested parties can achieve much. We hope that community rehabilitation will be seen as a valid field of research so that many of the unanswered questions can begin to be addressed.

In conclusion, for community rehabilitation to be successful we need to learn to integrate rehabilitation into the community and integrate the community into rehabilitation.

Index

Page numbers in *italics* refer to tables.